Evidence Based Counselling & Psychotherapy for the 21st Century Practitioner

Evidence Based Counselling & Psychotherapy for the 21st Century Practitioner

BY

DARYL MAHON

Outcomes Matter, Ireland

emerald
PUBLISHING

United Kingdom – North America – Japan – India – Malaysia – China

Emerald Publishing Limited
Howard House, Wagon Lane, Bingley BD16 1WA, UK

First edition 2023

British Library Cataloguing in Publication Data
A catalogue record for this book is available from the British Library

ISBN: 978-1-80455-733-4 (Print)
ISBN: 978-1-80455-732-7 (Online)
ISBN: 978-1-80455-734-1 (Epub)

Printed and bound by CPI Group (UK) Ltd, Croydon, CR0 4YY

ISOQAR certified Management System, awarded to Emerald for adherence to Environmental standard ISO 14001:2004.

Certificate Number 1985
ISO 14001

INVESTOR IN PEOPLE

Contents

List of Figures and Tables

Figures

Tables

Biographies

Author

Daryl Mahon, is a psychotherapist, lecturer and researcher. Prior to taking up his current role in research, he worked across the social inclusion sector, working with individuals and communities facing marginalisation. Much of his work has centred on substance use with people also involved in the criminal justice system, mental health difficulties and homelessness. More recently, he has been working as an Action Researcher with a European non-profit organisation based in Dublin working in complex systems change to support social services to solve complex problems and scale social innovations and evidence based practices.

He also lectures in Health and Social Care and delivers training to national and international practitioners and organisations. He has published in various peer reviewed areas related to psychotherapy processes and outcomes, trauma and leadership. His recently published best-selling book on Amazon, *Trauma Responsive Organisations: The Trauma Ecology Model* provides an in-depth exploration into trauma responsive organisations. He used the period during Covid to transition from psychotherapy practice to focus exclusively on research, training and lecturing.

Contributors

Jeb Brown completed his PhD in Counselling Psychology from Duke University in 1978. During the next two decades, he worked in a series of jobs where he was both a clinician and an administrator/supervisor, Including as Executive Director for The Center for Family Development, Executive Director of United Healthcare's Behavioural Health Systems in Utah and Director of Clinical Programmes for Aetna Health Plans. In 1998, he founded a consulting firm, the Center for Clinical Informatics, and began work on the ALERT Clinical Information System for PacifiCare Behavioural Health.

The ALERT system survived PacifiCare's acquisition by United Health Care and collaborative work with various academic researchers who were granted access to data within ALERT clinical information system resulted in a stream of peer reviewed articles advancing the methodology for benchmarking treatment outcomes. In 2007, he and Takuya Minami, PhD, founded the ACORN Collaboration and began work on a next generation clinical information system with a goal of greatly expanding the capabilities of older platforms. The Center for Clinical Informatics maintains the servers and programmes the system. The ACORN platform continues to build off lessons learned over 20 years of research and development, and regular use of the platform by practitioners has been demonstrated to measurably, clinically and meaningfully improve treatment outcomes from one year to the next. Until recently, he continues to maintain a part-time psychotherapy practice.

Ravind Jeawon, MIACP, is a licenced, Dublin-based psychotherapist and Founder of Talk Therapy Dublin, a service which aims to provide inclusive counselling supports to clients experiencing distress. His clinical experience began supporting community counselling services in Dublin providing psychotherapy and psychosocial support to communities affected by socioeconomic inequality, organised crime and homelessness. Having spent over three years in this area, he moved into private practice and noticed further demand by minoritised clients looking for responsive counselling linked to issues around ethnicity, race and the experience of migration. This encouraged an increasing interest in multiculturally responsive counselling, prompting him to pursue further training in the area at the Nafsiyat Intercultural Centre in London.

He has expanded his work to include training and the mentoring of students and newly qualified therapists from diverse backgrounds and provides counselling services to the International Organization for Migration in Ireland linked to their voluntary return programme. As a therapist, he continues to advocate for more inclusivity within mental health practice, particularly linked to core trainings and an improvement in multicultural responsiveness from caring professions when providing services to minoritised communities.

Ashley Simon, is a Co-owner of ACORN, a mental health analytics platform that tracks client progress and clinician effectiveness. Over her 10 years at ACORN, Ashley has worked as the head of Risk Assessment, QA, has co-authored on the collaboration's psychometric research, and now directs ACORN's content and training initiative. She holds a Master's degree in Middle East Studies and Linguistics, and a Bachelor's degree in Psychology.

Justin Turner, is a a Co-owner of ACORN. With over a decade of experience at ACORN as the operational manager, Justin oversees a wide array of daily functions. These functions include customer support, employee management and training, database management, form creation, and the creation of informational videos that help to inform clinicians of best practices for improving their clients' outcomes.

Acknowledgements

This is the second time in a 12-month period that I have sat down to write the acknowledgements part of a fully completed academic book. My reason for invoking this is not one of pride, although proud I am. The reason I bring this to the attention of the reader is to express my gratitude to my family, especially my wife. You don't write one, let alone two academic books during a 12-month period without the support of your family. To the unwavering support of my wife Jessica who puts up with my antics and long hours behind the computer screen, I love you. My children Zianna and Zayne, who never fail to enquire into my progress with my books. My hope is that I will be enquiring into the progress of both of your books in the future.

To my valued colleagues who contributed to chapters. Ravind Jeawon has come on board for the second time and brings his passion for making therapy more multiculturally responsive, thank you. To Dr Jeb Brown, who will be surprised to know that he helped plant the seed for this book, long before we ever met. Your contributions have greatly enriched this book and your life's work is truly impressive. It has been my absolute pleasure getting to know you during our online conversations and writing articles together.

Introduction

In the second year of my undergrad training in psychotherapy, two things happened that are relevant to the writing of this book. Firstly, I came across research on the common factors, and I read an article that was written by my now colleague, co-author and chapter contributor to this book, Dr Jeb Brown. Perhaps, I was put off by the response that the lecturer gave me when I brought the common factors up for discussion, or perhaps like the lecturer and many other practitioners, I didn't fully appreciate the relevance and significance of the common factors in therapy. Thus, my focus went elsewhere in the therapy literature. In psychotherapy, this generally means getting caught up in the next modality of therapy that is being marketed as the next great pill to solve a range of psychological issues. Unfortunately, much of psychotherapy research and practice likes to treat therapy like a medicine. That is, certain therapies work like a pill and act as remedial interventions for specific disorders or issues. Thankfully, it was not long before I was back on track and exploring the therapeutic factors that provide for effective psychotherapy, and it is these factors that make up a large part of this book. I seek to move the debate on by exploring what we know about the various factors (non-modalities) that contribute to the change process, and how we as a field can build on this knowledge through innovative deliberate practice training methods, and data-informed supervision.

I have always been curious as to how things work, no more so than with psychotherapy. So, as I delved back into the research on common factors and other aspects of psychotherapy processes and outcomes I was shocked to find that many of the criteria that we place huge value on have are generally not predictive of client outcomes. Years practicing, level of qualification, modality delivered, supervision, personal therapy, licencing body and continuing professional development do not tend to improve the effectiveness of the practitioner. I was both shocked and excited, and began to investigate these areas eagerly, publishing some papers. After spending many years practicing, researching and providing training in psychotherapy processes and outcomes, it makes sense to support this with an academic book. Whether you are a novice psychotherapy trainee, or a seasoned practitioner or supervisor, you will find this book a helpful evidence based resource. Over three sections, the chapters discuss evidence based practice in its various forms, including an analysis of research used, the debate around the effectiveness of specific therapies, commonalities across therapies and the many evidence based relationship variables that are said to contribute to effective psychotherapy. In addition, client factors are also discussed before moving onto exploring the use of technology, deliberate practice, supervision, and a simulated client case that will illustrate the application of some of the methods and ideas that we have outlined. As such, the book is structured across the following three sections, which describe what it is that an effective twenty-first century practitioner needs to know, do and reflect on to improve the effectiveness of their psychotherapeutic work and client outcomes.

Part 1

The first part of this book explores three key aspects of psychotherapy research and practice. In Chapter 1, I examine the evolution of empirically supported treatments (EST). Not without their criticism, I provide a historical perspective on EST and discuss how ESTs are often positioned as psychologies answer to medicine. That is, ESTs are treatments that are designed to reduce symptomology in the same way medicine provides a pill to treat a sick person. The role of the American Psychological Association in developing these therapies is outlined along with a critique of the role of the randomised control trial as a way to assess effectiveness of treatments.

In Chapter 2, I provide an overview of Evidence based practice (EBP) as defined and operationalised by the American Psychological Association. Crucially, in comparison to EST, EBP is positioned as a verb, as opposed to the noun like use of treatment modalities. The three components of EBP are discussed, namely:

1. The best available evidence; in conjunction with
2. Individual clinical expertise; that is consistent with
3. Client culture, values and preferences.

'Everyone has won, and all must have prizes'. This is the premise of the debate offered by the common factors proponents discussed in Chapter 3. The common factor debate rests on the idea that in general all treatment modalities will tend to be about equally effective because of non-specific treatment element that are common across diverse treatment approaches. It was Saul Rosenzweig in 1936 who first put forward the idea of commonalities among therapies. Since then, other researchers have built on these ideas, and this chapter tracks the trajectory of this research and the models proposed. The chapter finishes with some ideas regarding common and specific factors in therapy, ultimately, whether therapy gains its effectiveness from specific or common factors is perhaps a misleading dichotomy.

Part 2

The second section in this book deals with the substantive variables that have shown to impact on the outcome of psychotherapy. Altogether, I discuss 22 different factors that practitioners must consider under the heading of evidence based relationships, and evidence based responsiveness. In order to achieve this within the publishing guidelines, yet also provide the necessary information, a structured approach that provides a brief overview of each construct, along with the most up-to-date research, and the impact of the variable on psychotherapy outcomes is summarised. As such, the purpose is not to delve deep into each construct in detail, but rather, to provide a basic description to help the practitioner understand the variable being discussed, its empirical foundations and several top tips. The substantial bibliographies in each chapter will provide areas for further reading. Considering the breadth of constructs across this text, and given my aim to have this book act as a practical evidence based resource for the average practitioner to dip in and out of, having bite size chunks that practitioners can draw on is the best way to achieve this.

The first four chapters in Part 2 explore the research pertaining to evidence based relationships. Chapter 4 discusses the big impactful variables of the therapeutic alliance, goals and collaboration, alliance rupture–repair, and feedback-informed treatment. Chapter 5 explores how the idea of expectancy is conceptualised in psychotherapy, through treatment credibility and outcome expectancy, two key common factors that do not get discussed enough in the literature. Internal experiences can be considered to be the theme of Chapter 6, the relationship aspects of emotional expression, counter-transference, self-disclosure and immediacy are examined.

Finally, in Chapter 7, the big impactful variables of empathy, genuineness, unconditional positive regard and the real relationship are considered. Like previous chapters in this section, the research basis, impact and top tips are provided.

The second section of Part 2 focuses on evidence based responsiveness. While practitioners must be responsive to clients in various different ways, this part of the book provides an examination of responsiveness based on what we can consider to be client characteristics. In Chapter 8 and using the same format as in evidence based relationships, I set out the relevant research and impact of, attachment style, coping style, reactant level and stage of readiness for change Furthermore, the process of adapting treatment based on client preferences is considered. Multicultural responsiveness is dealt with in Chapter 9, Ravind Jeawon and I felt it necessary to have a whole chapter dedicated to this important area of psychotherapy practice. Ravind joins me once again to author a multicultural chapter, after co-authoring a chapter in my previous book on trauma responsive organisations.

Part 3

Part 3 of this book is where the idea of the twenty-first century practitioner really comes into its own. The final section of the book has four exciting chapters that will outline various innovative practices in the training and supervision of practitioners, in addition to the use of technology in therapy, and a simulated client case study demonstrating the application of many of the processes and practices discussed. I am grateful to have Dr Jeb Brown contribute Chapter 10 on the use of technology in psychotherapy. Anyone with an interest in the use of 'big data' for the purpose of psychotherapy will enjoy both the historic perspective, and the current innovations. Jeb also co-authored with me, a chapter on the use of data in supervision for the purpose of providing more effective care, and to inform deliberate practice.

Deliberate practice is a concept still in its infancy as applied to the initial training and ongoing continuous development of seasoned practitioners. Chapter 11 provides a rationale for the use of deliberate practice in the acquisition of psychotherapy skills and expertise. The processes and principles involved in this training regime are discussed, and I link it to the big impact variables outlined in the previous chapters as an initial method for skills acquisition. The use of routine outcome data in supervision is described in Chapter 12. Dr Jeb Brown and I provide the reader with picture of what the supervisory relationship in the twenty-first century can look like by using data to inform supervision and a deliberate practice training regime. Finally, Chapter 13 provides a simulated client case study for the twenty-first century practitioner and supervisor. A narrative commentary of a client–practitioner session illustrates the application of many of the variables discussed in this book, in addition to a practitioner–supervisor session focussed on using data and clinical information to inform supervision and deliberate practice to improve the acquisition of skills, and to enhance expertise and improve outcomes.

Part 1

Setting the Scene for Evidence Based Practice

Chapter 1

Empirically Supported Treatments: A Brief History

Daryl Mahon

Abstract

Psychotherapy is perhaps the most known and identifiable with one of the field's originators Sigmond Freud who is often accredited as being the inventor of the talking cure. However, it was many decades after psychoanalysis was first used by Freud that robust research and evidence was applied to psychotherapy, and its findings used to support practice in various contexts. While psychoanalysis is still practiced, the field has moved on and includes many hundreds if not thousands of approaches to healing. What has not improved, in general, is the between school rivalry regarding the efficacy and effectiveness of the different approaches. While it is now accepted that in general terms all approaches are about equally effective, certain research is often provided with more legitimacy than others. Mainly, the randomised control trial (RCT) is considered the gold standard in research terms, especially when it comes to establishing the efficacy and effectiveness of different psychotherapies. Empirically supported treatments (ESTs) are in prime position to take advantage of these political decisions, and this chapter will introduce the reader to these debates.

Keywords: Psychotherapy; empirically supported treatments; randomised control trial; evidence based practice; meta-analysis; evidence based treatments

Chapter Learning Outcomes

(1) Appreciate the historical application of research to psychotherapy practice.
(2) Introduce the reader to ESTs.

Evidence Based Counselling & Psychotherapy for the 21st Century Practitioner, 3–14

Published under exclusive licence by Emerald Publishing Limited
doi:10.1108/978-1-80455-732-720231001

Introduction

Psychotherapy is an effective treatment modality and has become a more professionalised service throughout the world. However, the research foundations for its efficacy are steeped in a long rivalry from within the profession. Competing theoretical orientations can be traced back to the Freudian era and are still very much in existence today. The claims of the superiority of one theory over another were a hot argument between Freud and his group, the therapy and practice of therapy was hotly and vehemently disputed. They were not alone, as the behaviourists joined the calls and criticised the analysts, while the humanistic theorists equally convinced of their approach provided a different way to view distress and healing. Behavioural ideas were incorporated into cognitive models and the third wave approaches sought alternative explanations. The next step of course was integrationist approaches which asked the question, 'what works for this person, delivered by that therapist?' The result is that there are now thousands of theories used to explain and treat human distress.

Norcross and Newman (1992, p. 3) provide the following analysis:

> Rivalry among theoretical orientations has a long and undistinguished history in psychotherapy, dating back to Freud. In the infancy of the field, therapy systems, like battling siblings, competed for attention and affection in a 'dogma eat dogma' environment .... Mutual antipathy and exchange of puerile insults between adherents of rival orientations were much the order of the day.

Emerging Research

Hans Eysenck (1952) in a review of the extant literature concluded that eclectic and psychoanalytic therapies were no more effective than no treatment at all. Controversy was to follow, with calls for potential clients to be informed of these findings on ethical grounds. In many respects, the within field fighting contributed to the lack of effectiveness of psychotherapeutic interventions being established within the research literature in the years to follow. This rivalry is not new. Going back to the earliest days of psychotherapy, we have seen how such rivalry split the various schools of psychoanalysis in the time of Freud and his colleagues.

Notwithstanding these issues, in time, the empirical support for psychotherapy began to emerge. Largely, this evidence was due to innovations in research power such as the RCT and the meta-analysis. RCTs are an experimental methodology where a person is randomly assigned to an active treatment, a control, or a waitlist to examine the effectiveness of the experiential treatment compared to another control (Wampold, 2013), as such, casual inferences can then be drawn. During the 1970s, hundreds of such studies had been carried out confirming the effectiveness of psychotherapy, regardless of the type of approach to treatment (Bergin, 1971), these studies of equivalence as they are known, have been replicated throughout the literature (Leonidaki & Constantinou, 2022; Stiles et al., 2008; Wampold et al., 2017; Watts et al., 2013). However, it was the emergence of the meta-analysis that allowed studies to be pooled together to give an overall effect size for psychological therapies, and this method demonstrated the field's prowess.

The meta-analysis brings together similar studies that are often relatively homogenous and pools together their effect sizes and reports on overall effectiveness. A seminal study (Smith & Glass, 1977) utilised this statistical analysis to review 375 studies and found that the average treated person was more better off than 60–82% of those receiving no treatment. In the years since Eysenck's (1952) claims that psychotherapeutic practices were not effective healing agents, much has been debated. Discourses have evolved, shifted, and reflected on several key debates. We now know that psychotherapy is an effective treatment modality (Lambert, 2013; Lambert & Ogles, 2004; Wampold & Imel, 2015). In fact, therapists in naturalistic settings reach the often cited 0.80 effect size benchmark from highly controlled RCTs (Wampold & Imel, 2015). Hence, psychotherapy has been established as an effective treatment modality on par with some medical treatments such as heart bypass surgery and chemotherapy for breast cancer (Lipsey & Wilson, 1993). Indeed, this is not where the comparison to the medical model ends, controversy around ESTs based within a medical paradigm of specific treatments for specific disorders is a hot topic within the psychotherapeutic discourse and has an interesting history.

Specific Ingredients

Specific ingredients refer to those aspects of a treatment modality that are proposed to be the mechanisms of change. With regard to research, most studies examining specific factors in therapies have done so through cognitive behavioural therapy (CBT) and anxiety and depression. In a review of 30 meta-analyses, Kazantzis et al. (2018) synthesised the outcome process with regard to CBT, largely within the treatment of anxiety and depression. They found the strongest support for cognitive and behavioural strategies as processes of change in depression and anxiety. In another meta-analysis that included 35 studies, Lemmens, Müller, Arntz, and Huibers (2016) examined the mechanisms of change in CBT and other therapies. The strongest findings from this review support mechanisms of change related to negative automatic thoughts, dysfunctional attitudes, worry, rumination, and the use of mindfulness.

Using 26 studies, Cristea et al. (2015) performed a meta-analysis of the effects of CBT on dysfunctional thinking, which is often suggested to be the core process in CBT. However, when compared to other psychotherapies in the study, there was no significant differences, which could mean that dysfunctional thinking is not exclusive to CBT. Spinhoven et al. (2018) conducted a meta-analysis of 36 studies that investigated the effects of various forms of CBT on repetitive negative thinking compared with various other treatment types. They found significantly larger effect sizes for CBT treatments such as rumination-focussed CBT and original CBT compared with treatments such as antidepressant medication and counselling. When thinking about these studies, it is important to realise that much of the evidence is correlational, and that we are still not at a point where we are carrying out the type of complex research needed to draw inferences about causality. As Cuijpers, Reijnders, and Huibers (2019) suggest, 'evidence for the mediational role of the various constructs (specific and non-specific) is largely mixed and that better designed studies are urgently needed to understand the mechanisms of psychotherapy'. However, as we will see in subsequent chapters, we may have arrived at a point where we can draw inferences about causality as it relates to the therapeutic alliance.

The Road to ESTs

Evidence based practice (EBP) within the counselling and psychotherapy professions can be traced back to the evidence based medicine movement. Leff (2002) informs us of three key issues that influenced the medical field and the promotion of this paradigm.

(1) Reforms of physician training in 1910 lead to a call for curriculum to be underpinned by science.
(2) In 1948, the *British Medical Journal* published what was the first RCT.
(3) The final influence was the creation of the Food and Drug Administration agency and the double blind RCT, which is considered the gold standard research trial for establishing efficacies' interventions.

Throughout the 1990s evidence based medicine was further integrated into the system based on the work of people like Archi Cochrane and David Sackett, with the former being influential in embedding the RCT as the standard for evidence based interventions, and the latter being one of the driving forces behind articulating and conceptualising EBP in medicine. At the same time that Sackett and colleagues were moving to an evidence-practice paradigm in medicine, psychiatry through the American Psychiatric Association were attempting to categorise and promote practice guidelines across discrete 'disorders'. However, in contrast to what was occurring in medicine, psychiatrists' evidence of a biological basis was non-existent, and was exclusively based on consensus between those 'around the table'. With the subsequent treatments derived from these decisions. Thus, psychiatry went about legitimising their approach to mental health not through a scientific paradigm but based on consensus between practitioners (Duncan & Reese, 2012).

Concurrently, psychologists rushed to find methods to counter psychiatry's magic pills, establishing ESTs. In what has been described by Duncan and Reese (2012) as 'perhaps fearing psychiatry's historical hegemony in health care' ESTs were promoted as a 'common cause' for a clinical profession fighting exclusion'. Suggesting that care should be 'proven', not consensus treatments, a special task force (Chambless, 1993) acting under the auspices of American Psychological Association (APA) Division 12 (Society of Clinical Psychology) set forth its conclusions about what constituted scientifically valid treatments. Drawing on the concept of evidence based medicine, and on the idea that the quality of client care is improved when practitioners use treatments with empirical support as noted by Sackett, Richardson, Rosenberg, and Haynes (2000), the Task Force first selected a set of criteria by which to identify the presence of adequate scientific evidence. Thus, the Task Force concentrated its efforts on research demonstrating that a particular treatment has proven to be beneficial for clients in RCTs and based their categorisation of these therapies under three headings: strong, modest, and controversial. The Task Force reviewed available research and catalogued treatments of choice for specific diagnoses based on their efficacy criteria, in the same manner as the US Food and Drug Administration before them. To date, a list of over 80 ESTs for 27 of the 157 diagnoses in the *DSM-5* have been created, which, as far as outcomes are concerned, has done little by the way of improving therapist effectiveness (Schukard, Miller, & Hubble, 2017).

Empirically Supported Treatments

What do we mean when we refer to ESTs? Therapies that can be manualised, with supposedly specific ingredients for specific 'disorders' based on the medical model paradigm of symptom reduction (Norcross & Wampold, 2019). As Shean (2016, p. 1) posits:

> RCT studies favour therapies that focus on specific symptoms and can be described in a manual, administered reliably across patients, completed in relatively few sessions, and involve short-term evaluations of outcome.

ESTs can be found by their abbreviated names. For example, Dialectal Behaviour Therapy, Acceptance and Commitment Therapy among others. Importantly, ESTs have the following characteristics, they are: manualised treatments based on protocols; delivered with fidelity; have supposedly specific ingredients; used for specific presenting issues, and are short-term interventions. The following research criteria (adapted from Tolin, McKay, Forman, Klonsky, & Thombs, 2015) are needed to assess if ESTs are considered well established and probably effective.

(A) At least two good between-group design experiments demonstrating efficacy in one or more of the following ways:

   (1) Superior (based on statistical significance alone) to pill or psychological placebo or to another treatment.

(2) Equivalent to an already established treatment in experiments with adequate statistical power, considered to be approximately 30 per group.

(B) A large series of single-case design experiments ($n > 9$) demonstrating efficacy. These experiments must have:

(1) Used good experimental designs.
(2) Compared the intervention to another treatment as in A.1.

Further criteria for both (A) and (B) are as follows:

(1) Experiments must be conducted with treatment manuals.
(2) Characteristics of the client samples must be clearly specified.
(3) Effects must have been demonstrated by at least two different investigators or investigating teams.

For the American Psychological Association (2002, p. 1054).

> Randomized controlled experiments represent a more stringent way to evaluate treatment efficacy because they are the most effective way to rule out threats to internal validity in a single experiment.

However, this position has various major flaws. For example, unlike in medicine where the RCT rains supreme, in therapy it is impossible to have a double-blind study, or even a single blind for that matter. How would we blind either the therapist to the type of treatment they are providing, or the client who is receiving therapy? In medicine, this is achieved by providing the patient with a placebo pill, in therapy this is not possible. Thus, in therapy research, treatment manuals are used, therapists are trained in their use, internal validity is maintained, and the therapist themselves are not deemed important. However, as we will see in further chapters, the therapist is perhaps the biggest variable in the treatment process and attempting to control the therapist as an unimportant variable is not the correct approach to take.

As we can see, ESTs are put forward in the same way that psychiatry uses certain pills for certain ills, however, as we will see later, psychotherapy is nothing like psychiatry, and disorder specific treatments may not be the gold standard approach that prevails when they are compared to another valid/bona fide treatment approaches. Controversy remains, with some advocates positing that ESTs are no more effective than the hundreds of other theoretical approaches within the field (Sakaluk, Williams, Kilshaw, & Rhyner, 2019). Further, Tackett and Miller (2019) and Sakaluk et al. (2019) call into question the actual evidence for ESTs, issues of methodology in RCTs, such as comparing treatments to control groups receiving no treatment, and issues with a lack of replication that are widespread. Another research suggests that ESTs don't always transition into naturalistic settings due to controls utilised to improve internal validity during RCTs. Real world practice is often very different than research trials, where client's characteristics and therapist factors are kept consistent. Thus, this research evidence is often inconsistent with the average practitioners' experience in real settings (Margison et al., 2000).

Despite the concerns about the use of RCTs to investigation psychotherapy, and as noted above, in 1995, a Task Force within Clinical Psychology of the APA, reviewed the evidence obtained in RCTs and generated a list of treatments that, in their opinion, had achieved an appropriate level of empirical support and could put psychotherapy on an equal playing field with its main competitor, psychiatry (Schuckard, Miller, & Hubble, 2017). With each new diagnosis or topical issue, a new set of treatments are put forward as empirically supported, which has ramifications politically as far as treatment issues such as policy, reimbursement, and practice are concerned. This can be seen in the latest treatment guidelines for the treatment of trauma. The APA continues to promulgate the EST proposition and recently produced a controversial (Norcross & Wampold, 2019) clinical guidelines with a rating category for specific trauma treatments. Norcross and Wampold (2019) critique these guidelines and suggest that there are no clinically meaningful difference between the Strongly Recommended and Conditionally Recommend therapies. Thankfully, this is not a one-sided story, and while the RCT is still considered the gold standard, other bodies within the APA, notably Division 29, were voicing concerns regarding the level of importance given to the treatment method, when other variables have as much as, and often more impact on treatment outcomes. The next chapters on EBP, and the common factors will unpack this debate further, and introduce the reader to a wider conceptualisation of EBP and provide an overview of the differential variables that contribute to effective outcomes in psychological therapies.

While there is nothing inherently wrong in providing ESTs, wider treatment factors need to be considered, especially those that have as much as or often more impact on the outcome of counselling and psychotherapy. Lest we not forget, one cannot gain EST status if the treatment cannot be manualised and studied in a RCT. This becomes problematic when policy makers and systems of care give priority to ESTs, commissioning bodies, insurance companies, and other stakeholders often mandate practitioners to use 'evidence based' therapies.

> Recent proposals to adopt policies that dictate training, credentialing, and reimbursement based on lists of EBTs unduly limit how psychotherapy can be conceptualized and practiced and are not in the best interests of the profession or of individuals seeking psychotherapy services. (Shean, 2016, p. 45)

While this system is most pronounced in America, England has followed suit with the National Institute for Health and Care Excellence (NICE) guidelines. NICE is not without its critics either and the Improving Access to Psychological Therapies programme (largely CBT) has been critiqued as not being more effective than other therapies (Leonidaki, 2019; McPherson et al., 2018). Other international providers are also following this trajectory, with the hegemony of the RCT and manualised therapies often being provided with the leading voice in policy decisions. In a meta-review of the EST literature, Sakaluk et al. (2019) made the following evaluation, which indicates that the position adapted with regard to these treatments may not be the whole picture:

> Empirically supported treatments ... are the gold standard in therapeutic interventions for psychopathology. Based on a set of methodological and statistical criteria, the APA has assigned particular treatment-diagnosis combinations EST status and has further rated their empirical support as Strong, Modest, and/or Controversial. Emerging concerns about the replicability of research findings in clinical psychology highlight the need to critically examine the evidential value of EST research .... Our analyses indicated that power and replicability estimates were concerningly low across almost all ESTs, and individually, some ESTs scored poorly across multiple metrics, with Strong ESTs failing to continuously outperform their Modest counterparts.

Various issues have been highlighted in the use of ESTs. In particular, the use of the RCT and the many flaws, not all of which have been outlined here. Research power due to advancements in methodology has improved in the 30 years since the criteria for ESTs were first articulated. We now have much more powerful studies and evidence synthesis that can be used to inform policy and practice decisions for therapeutic interventions. For example, systematic reviews and meta-analyses discussed earlier in this chapter are much better suited methods to base decisions on the weight of evidence they can produce based on the inclusion of multiple studies with many more participants. While these syntheses will include RCTs, they will do so at a level that can draw conclusion about the strength of evidence provided in each individual study, meaning biases can be accounted for with more transparency. One of the other strong criticisms of the process of evidence generation of RCTs and ESTs is that the intervention only needs to demonstrate to be effective in two studies, and as such, other null or negative findings are not considered. This of course is problematic when we consider research bias and allegiance. Evidence synthesis is one way to counteract some of these challenges. In Table 1, I chart some of the concerns and possible solutions to these problems.

Table 1. Areas of Concern and Some Solutions.

Treatment Issues	Criticism	Moving Forward
Reliability of findings from studies	• Differences often found in the effectiveness of studies using same treatments	• The use of and effectiveness of treatments should be based on evidence synthesis (Cochrane review/meta-analyses), especially where policy/guidelines are making treatment recommendations or categorising the effectiveness of treatments
	• Statistical significance is not a measure of effectiveness	• Treatments should be assessed by their clinical significance in addition to statistical significance
	• No weight given to negative outcomes	• Qualitative methods should be used to help understand negative findings
	• Relative effectiveness not considered enough	• Decisions to use treatments should include the effectiveness of a treatment relative to other treatments, not inactive controls
Validity of findings	• Treatments struggle to generalise to non-research settings with the same effectiveness	• Treatment studies should be conducted in real world settings, in addition to efficacy studies
	• Differences between individual practitioners (therapists effects) not accounted for	• Therapist effects should be controlled for in all studies
	• Fidelity to protocols does not generalise into routine practice	• Protocols should be used flexibly in treatment settings
Specificity of treatments	• Concerns around specific ingredients as mechanism of change	• More dismantling studies should be used more to assess if specific ingredients are causing change
	• Treatments focussed on symptom reduction only	• Symptom reduction should be replaced with measures of global change to include functioning and other important psychosocial outcomes

Conclusion

Psychotherapy has a long and often rivalrous history, with competing theoretical orientations being positioned as the magic pill. Indeed, much of the current ideas around specificity can be traced back to psychologies desire to be placed on an equal footing with psychiatry. No doubt research power has improved since the time when Hans Eysenck's claims were disputed. However, whether ESTs provide any additional meaningful benefit over their counterparts is still hotly disputed. In the following chapter, I introduce the reader to EBP as a concept with a wider remit than just the treatment modality.

References

American Psychological Association. (2002). Criteria for evaluating treatment guidelines. *American Psychologist*, *57*, 1052–1059.

Chambless, D. L. (1993). Task force on promotion and dissemination of psychological procedures: A report adopted by the Division 12 Board-October 1993.

Cristea, I. A., Huibers, M. J., David, D., Hollon, S. D., Andersson, G., & Cuijpers, P. (2015). The effects of cognitive behavior therapy for adult depression on dysfunctional thinking: A meta-analysis. *Clinical Psychology Review*, *42*, 62–71. https://doi.org/10.1016/j.cpr.2015.08.003

Cuijpers, P., Reijnders, M., & Huibers, M. (2019). The role of common factors in psychotherapy outcomes. *Annual Review of Clinical Psychology*, *15*, 207–231. https://doi.org/10.1146/annurev-clinpsy-050718-095424

Duncan, B. L., & Reese, R. J. (2012). Empirically supported treatments, evidence-based treatments, and evidence-based practice. In I. Weiner, G. Stricker, & T. A. Widiger (Eds.), *Handbook of psychology* (2nd ed.). https://doi.org/10.1002/9781118133880.hop208021

Eysenck, H. J. (1952). The effects of psychotherapy: An evaluation. *Journal of Consulting Psychology*, *16*(5), 319–324. https://doi.org/10.1037/h0063633

Garfield, S. L., & Bergin, A. E. (1971). Personal therapy, outcome and some therapist variables. *Psychotherapy: Theory, Research & Practice*, *8*(3), 251–253. https://doi.org/10.1037/h0086667

Kazantzis, N., Luong, H. K., Usatoff, A. S., Impala, T., Yew, R. Y., & Hofmann, S. G. (2018). The processes of cognitive behavioral therapy: A review of meta-analyses. *Cognitive Therapy and Research*, *42*, 349–357.

Lambert, M. J. (2013). Outcome in psychotherapy: The past and important advances. *Psychotherapy*, *50*(1), 42–51. https://doi.org/10.1037/a0030682

Lambert, M. J. & Ogles, B. M. (2004). The efficacy and effectiveness of psychotherapy. In M. J. Lambert's (Ed.), *Bergin and Garfield's handbook of psychotherapy and behavior Change* (pp. 139–193). New York: Wiley.

Leff, H. S. (2002). *A brief history of evidence-based practice*. Mental Health.

Lemmens, L. H., Müller, V. N., Arntz, A., & Huibers, M. J. (2016). Mechanisms of change in psychotherapy for depression: An empirical update and evaluation of research aimed at identifying psychological mediators. *Clinical Psychology Review*, *50*, 95–107.

Leonidaki, V. (2019). Moving beyond a single-model philosophy: Integrating relational therapies in front-line psychological therapy services in England. *Journal of Psychotherapy Integration*, *31*(1), 70–85. https://doi.org/10.1037/int0000192

Leonidaki, V., & Constantinou, M. P. (2022). A comparison of completion and recovery rates between first-line protocol-based cognitive behavioural therapy and non-manualized relational therapies within a UK psychological service. *Clinical Psychology & Psychotherapy*, *29*(2), 754–766. https://doi.org/10.1002/cpp.2669

Lipsey, M., & Wilson, D. (1993). The efficacy of psychological, educational, and behavioral treatment: Confirmation from meta-analyses. *American Psychologist*, *48*, 1181–1209.

Margison, F. R., Barkham, M., Evans, C., McGrath, G., Clark, J. M., Audin, K., & Connell, J. (2000). Measurement and psychotherapy. Evidence-based practice and practice-based evidence. *The British Journal of Psychiatry: The Journal of Mental Science*, *177*, 123–130. https://doi.org/10.1192/bjp.177.2.123

McPherson, S., Rost, F., Town, J., & Abbass, A. (2018). Epistemological flaws in NICE review methodology and its impact on recommendations for psychodynamic psychotherapies for complex and persistent depression. *Psychoanalytic Psychotherapy*, *32*(2), 102–121.

Norcross, J. C., & Newman, C. F. (1992). Psychotherapy integration: Setting the context. In J. C. Norcross & M. R. Goldfried (Eds.), *Handbook of psychotherapy integration* (pp. 3–45). New York, NY: Basic Books.

Norcross, J. C., & Wampold, B. E. (2019). Relationships and responsiveness in the psychological treatment of trauma: The tragedy of the APA Clinical Practice Guideline. *Psychotherapy*, *56*(3), 391–399. https://doi.org/10.1037/pst0000228

Sackett, D., Richardson, S., Rosenberg, W., & Haynes, B. (2000). *Evidence based medicine: How to practice and teach EBM*. London: Churchill Livingstone.

Sakaluk, J. K., Williams, A. J., Kilshaw, R. E., & Rhyner, K. T. (2019). Evaluating the evidential value of empirically supported psychological treatments (ESTs): A meta-scientific review. *Journal of Abnormal Psychology*, *128*(6), 500–509. https://doi.org/10.1037/abn0000421

Schuckard, E., Miller, S. D., & Hubble, M. A. (2017). Feedback-informed treatment: Historical and empirical foundations. In D. S. Prescott, C. L. Maeschalck, & S. D. Miller (Eds.), *Feedback-informed treatment in clinical practice: Reaching for excellence* (pp. 13–35). Washington, DC: American Psychological Association.

Shean, G. (2016). Psychotherapy outcome research: Issues and questions. *Psychodynamic Psychiatry*, *44*(1), 1–24. https://doi.org/10.1521/pdps.2016.44.1.1

Smith, M. L., & Glass, G. V. (1977). Meta-analysis of psychotherapy outcome studies. *American Psychologist*, *32*(9), 752–760.

Spinhoven, P., Klein, N., Kennis, M., Cramer, A., Siegle, G., Cuijpers, P., … Bockting, C. L. (2018). The effects of cognitive-behavior therapy for depression on repetitive negative thinking: A meta-analysis. *Behaviour Research and Therapy*, *106*, 71–85. https://doi.org/10.1016/j.brat.2018.04.002

Stiles, W. B., Barkham, M., Mellor-Clark, J., & Connell, J. (2008). Effectiveness of cognitive-behavioural, person-centred, and psychodynamic therapies in UK primary-care routine practice: Replication in a larger sample. *Psychological Medicine*, *38*(5), 677–688. https://doi.org/10.1017/S0033291707001511

Tackett, J. L., & Miller, J. D. (2019). Introduction to the special section on increasing replicability, transparency, and openness in clinical psychology. *Journal of Abnormal Psychology*, *128*(6), 487–492. https://doi.org/10.1037/abn0000455

Tolin, D. F., McKay, D., Forman, E. M., Klonsky, E. D., & Thombs, B. D. (2015). Empirically supported treatment: Recommendations for a new model. *Clinical Psychology: Science and Practice*, *22*(4), 317–338. https://doi.org/10.1037/h0101729

Wampold, B. E. (2013). The good, the bad, and the ugly: A 50-year perspective on the outcome problem. *Psychotherapy*, *50*(1), 16–24. https://doi.org/10.1037/a0030570

Wampold, B. E., Baldwin, S. A., Holtforth, M. G., & Imel, Z. E. (2017). What characterizes effective therapists? In L. G. Castonguay & C. E. Hill (Eds.), *How and why are some therapists better than others?: Understanding therapist effects* (pp. 37–53). Washington, DC: American Psychological Association. https://doi.org/10.1037/0000034-003

Wampold, B. E., & Imel, Z. E. (2015). (2nd ed.). London: Routledge/Taylor & Francis Group.

Watts, B. V., Schnurr, P. P., Mayo, L., Young-Xu, Y., Weeks, W. B., & Friedman, M. J. (2013). Meta-analysis of the efficacy of treatments for posttraumatic stress disorder. *The Journal of Clinical Psychiatry*, *74*(6), e541–e550. https://doi.org/10.4088/JCP.12r08225

Chapter 2

Evidence Based Practice: An Overview

Daryl Mahon

Abstract

In the last chapter, I introduced the reader to the concept of empirically supported treatments and some of the research methods of providing evidence for the effectiveness of these interventions. Unfortunately, the field seems to place much importance on the techniques and methods used by the practitioner, when the reality is that there are a vast amount of components and variables that contribute to change in effective psychotherapy. In this chapter, I move beyond the idea of the treatment method and explore the idea of evidence based practice (EBP) in its entirety. The reader will be provided with a description of EBP as a tripartite model. While it is beyond the current chapter to delve in depth into each aspect of EBP, the chapter does act as an excellent introduction providing the practitioner with key learnings to build on.

Keywords: Evidence based practice; American Psychological Association; clinical expertise; psychotherapy; counselling; best practice

Chapter Learning Outcomes

(1) Describe EBP.
(2) Understand how the components of EBP interact and the implications for treatment.

Introduction

In the previous chapter, I provided a historical trajectory of psychotherapy research and introduced the reader to the idea of empirically supported treatments. In this chapter, we are going to move beyond the idea of the treatment

Evidence Based Counselling & Psychotherapy for the 21st Century Practitioner, 15–25

Published under exclusive licence by Emerald Publishing Limited
doi:10.1108/978-1-80455-732-720231002

method/theory and examine how EBP is conceptualised, while discussing its various components. It is vitally important for practitioners to recognise and understand their craft, in all its glory. However, much debate, research, and practice tends to stay at the level of the treatment method. Unfortunately, for both practitioners and clients alike, this narrow view only serves to miss the richness of counselling and psychotherapy components, and make the practice of counselling and psychotherapy less effective.

Both EBP and the latest guidelines for practice set out by the American Psychological Association (APA, 2021) will be discussed. While there are many different institutes that regulate and support the practice of therapy, The APA are more established with many different divisions and are thus considered leaders in the field of counselling and psychotherapy. As such, much of their work can be considered instructional for practitioners as it is well researched and based on meta-analyses by key thinkers and researchers in the field.

Evidence Based Guidelines

Very recently, the APA (2021) produced a guiding document for practitioner and those involved in the training of those who practice counselling and psychotherapy: The APA Practice Guidelines on Evidenced Based Practice in Healthcare (Table 2). The report puts forward nine guidelines for practitioners to engage in based on a substantial review and synthesise of evidence. As many of these practice guidelines have been assimilated from the concept of EBP, and indeed the practice guidelines themselves have EBP in the guidelines, we will largely focus on a discussion of, and the operationalisation of EBP and its implications for therapeutic practitioners.

Table 2. Guidelines from APA.

Guideline 1	Psychologists are mindful of the principles and importance of EBP
Guideline 2	Psychologists strive to maintain and enhance their knowledge of the research and scholarly literature applicable to their practice
Guideline 3	Psychologists endeavour to conduct assessments that are appropriate for the setting, purpose, and population
Guideline 4	Psychologists seek to participate in collaborative treatment planning with patients and others when appropriate.
Guideline 5	Psychologists aim to cultivate and maintain effective therapeutic relationships, therapist characteristics, and change principles
Guideline 6	Psychologists will adapt their clinical approach to patient characteristics, culture, and preferences in ways that increase effectiveness

Table 2. (*Continued*)

Guideline 7	Psychologists aim to monitor the treatment process and clinical outcomes routinely
Guideline 8	Psychologists seek to modify their clinical approach when appropriate and terminate treatment when the patient is no longer benefitting or when treatment goals have been met

According the APA (2006), EBP consists of the integration of the best available research, with clinical expertise in the context of the client's characteristics, culture, and preferences. As we can see with this definition, while treatment methods may be one aspect, there are various other components that need to be considered under the EBP concept. As we can see the conceptualisation of EBP is closely aligned to that proposed in evidence based medicine discussed in the previous chapter (Sackett, Straus, Richardson, Rosenberg, & Haynes, 2000). I will provide a summary of this tripartite model (Fig. 1) under the heading of the three components.

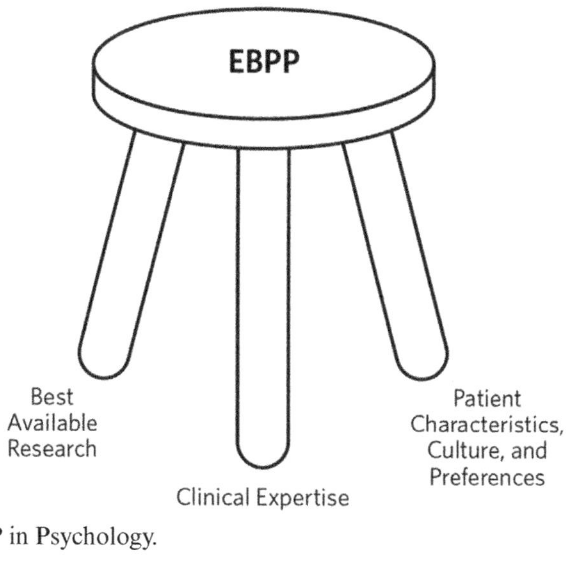

Fig. 1. EBP in Psychology.

Best Available Research Evidence

In many ways, in the previous chapter, I have indicated the type and the scope of evidence that are considered the gold standard in therapy research. However, these methodologies are not without their limitations, as have all methods to the collection and interpretation of data. While this section is far from an exhaustive list, the following are discussed by the APA (2006) under the best available research heading. That is, the types of evidence it deems necessary to base clinical decisions on. Various types of research can be used. Table 3 illustrates these methodologies.

Table 3. Types of Research Used to Establish Effectiveness of Psychological Therapies.

Type of Study	Explanation
Clinical observations	Observations in clinical practice and the use of single case studies can lead to practitioners generating hypotheses and resulting innovations, and are considered the most rudimentary psychological science
Qualitative methods	Qualitative research can provide rich descriptions of how an intervention works, or doesn't work by drawing on the lived experience of participants
Aggregated case studies	Used across networks can be very useful for describing characteristics of individuals and interventions in practice contexts
Ethnographic research	Can be helpful across organisational or other contexts to establish if interventions are acceptable, effective, their availability, or for making recommendation on their utility or need for adapting them to a given context or characteristic
Process–outcome studies	Can be useful for establishing mechanisms of change in various interventions, for example, dismantling studies, or studies examining variables and their relationship to outcomes
RCT	RCTs are used to draw conclusions on causality, efficacy, and effectiveness of interventions, based on the randomisation of people to interventions being tested in experimental designs
Meta-analysis	Are a type of evidence synthesis, where many RCTs are pooled together to answer a question about effectiveness while also exploring possible mediators and mediators of the interventions and evidence quality. Overall effectiveness is reported as a Cohen's *d* effect size

Source: Adapted from APA (2006).

Best available research is understood to mean different types of evidence related to psychosocial interventions, assessment processes and strategies, clinical presentations, and varied populations (APA, 2006). At the same time, research needs to provide balance between internal and external validity, and as I discussed in the previous chapter, the RCT in controlled settings is largely focussed on internal validity, meaning external validity (interventions in natural settings) may not have the same effectiveness as original trials. Other issues that also need to be considered, include what weight should be given to sample size and power of the study; representation and issues of diversity; generalisability and utility;

and mechanisms of proposed change, comparisons used in trials, and the significance of findings. Thus, no one research approach will be able to capture all these factors and drawing on meta-analysis or several meta-analyses may be needed when it comes to policy or commissioning decisions.

However, as I discussed in the previous chapter, the default position by many is the RCT as it is provided with the gold standard label for conducting intervention trials. While the RCT can be a valuable method, in many psychotherapy studies it is used in have serious issues with their methodologies, including in those studies that pool results, the meta-analysis (Dragioti, Dimoliatis, & Evangelou, 2015; Wampold & Serlin, 2014). Moreover, researcher allegiance in comparison studies is said to account for a significant amount of treatment effects (Munder, Flückiger, Gerger, Wampold, & Barth, 2012). At the same time, a meta-analytic review of researcher allegiance suggests that very few researchers (0.2%) put in place procedures to account for its impact on their study findings (Dragioti et al., 2015).

Although the APA (2006) outline the usefulness of differentiated research methods, when it comes to policy on interventions, the following position taken from the Criteria for Evaluating Treatment Guidelines (APA, 2002, p. 1053) is more suited to the RCT.

> The first dimension is treatment efficacy, the systematic and scientific evaluation of whether a treatment works. The second dimension is clinical utility, the applicability, feasibility, and usefulness of the intervention in the local or specific setting where it is to be offered. This dimension also includes determination of the generalizability of an intervention whose efficacy has been established.

Of course, treatment efficacy is important as an initial first stage of intervention development, however, interventions are tightly controlled in these studies by the use of protocols, as are the characteristics of the people being provided with the interventions. We referred to this earlier as internal validity. That is, the study is giving itself the best opportunity under the best condition to demonstrate its effectiveness. However, as the average practitioner will testify, conditions in routine practice are far from perfect, indeed, depending on the context, setting and population you are working with, things can be a lot different. Clients will often have more than one presenting problem and various other factors that impact on therapy, including that of the therapist (Johns, Barkham, Kellett, & Saxon, 2019; Wampold & Brown, 2005), the client (Norcross, 2002; Wampold & Imel, 2015), and the setting (Firth, Saxon, Stiles, & Barkham, 2019) and may be extremely different than that in the RCT where the intervention was first evaluated. Thus, the second dimension of clinical utility (applicability, feasibility, and usefulness) needs to be assessed in the various contexts that the intervention is to be applied in.

Clinical utility includes various components such as the applicability of the intervention, the acceptance of the intervention by the populations it has been designed for, and the generalisability of the intervention across settings and clients. For example, an intervention studied in trials that included mainly White Western populations cannot be assumed to be effective outside of this demographic, nor can an intervention that has shown to be effective working with one issue assumed to be effective with another. For example, an intervention that has demonstrated to be effective with anxiety cannot be assumed to be effective with depression, from evidence based perspective, at least.

The utility and the feasibility of the intervention are another criteria to consider. An intervention can have really strong evidence behind it, but if it is difficult to bring it into real world settings, if its use is too costly, and practitioners and clients find it burdensome, then it will be difficult to implement in routine practice. Again, the RCT can be used to answer some of these questions. However, increasingly, it is being recognised that mixed methods, with an RCT and a qualitative methodology, that seeks to understand the why and how of an intervention is necessary when it comes to implementation and investigating its utility and brevity. As such, a well-designed meta-analysis that provides evidence of the effectiveness of an intervention, compared to another active control, that also provides research on the acceptability, clinical utility, and applicability is perhaps the best type of research that a practitioner can use to make clinical decisions. Of course, these clinical decisions cannot be made in isolation and need to consider client characteristics and preferences, that is, through the use of clinical expertise.

Clinical Expertise

Clinical expertise from an EBP perspective is not a term utilised to describe top preforming practitioners. Rather it is used to denote the experience gained throughout training and education, continuous development, and practices engaged in that contribute to competency development across the life of the practitioner's development (APA, 2006). As such, clinical expertise has many components and is also context specific. At the same time, context is only one small element as the components of clinical expertise are also largely trans-theoretical. That is, they cross the different types of practice and trainings provided to practitioners.

Clinical expertise allows practitioners to operationalise the EBP model, as it were. It achieves this because clinical expertise contributes to the understanding of how to integrate the best available research with the third element of EBP, client characteristics, culture, and preferences within the context of the treatment process (APA, 2021). As I noted previously, the treatment provider accounts for more of the variance in change than the actual treatment method, as such, it is paramount to have a sound knowledge and clinical expertise. The following guidelines adapted from the APA can be instructional for practitioners when considering their scope of clinical expertise, and in planning their continuous development and education. As the reader will appreciate, each of these eight areas are generic, however, they can also be applied in a context-specific manner, depending on the construct, setting, or population a practitioner is working in.

Assessment, Diagnostic Judgement, Systematic Case Formulation, and Treatment Planning. Assessment and psychological assessment are used in a collaborative manner by practitioners and clients to gather information about the issues clients would like to seek support for. Assessment helps to clarify presenting issues, assess treatment preferences (Swift, Callahan, Cooper, & Parkin, 2018), and client characteristics, and for some practitioners to make diagnoses of psychological 'disorders' such as anxiety or depression (Beck, Epstein, Brown, & Steer, 1988; Beck, Ward, Mendelson, Mock, & Erbaugh, 1961), or indeed to assess attachment style, or stage of change. Assessment is also used to inform treatment planning, case conceptualisation, and goal setting. Assessment occurs from initial intake and includes the administration of standardised instruments to assess psychological processes, to monitor the experience of the client (therapeutic alliance), and evaluate the benefit (outcomes) of care (Brown, Simon, Cameron, & Minami, 2015). Practitioners also make use of their judgement and assess clients informally throughout therapy using open-ended questions and reflection. This is especially important when using standardised measures, practitioners must use all information available to them, and information derived from formal assessment must be used within the practitioner's scope of practice, including their clinical decision-making abilities.

Case conceptualisation is the use of assessment information to explain and develop responses to the presenting issues based on best research evidence, theoretical concepts, and the client's narrative and input. Case conceptualisation seeks to examine and explain presenting problems by describing factors that contribute to distress, how clients respond to this distress, and strengths that can be used to help alleviate distress. Practitioners will use this information to choose interventions and strategies that they know have evidence and will best fit the situation.

Treatment planning is a process that involves moving from the 'problem to the solution' The APA (2006, p. 276) suggest that:

> Treatment planning involves setting goals and tasks of treatment that take into consideration the unique patient, the nature of the patient's problems and concerns, the likely prognosis and expected benefits of treatment, and available resources.

As we will see later in this book, collaborative goal work contributes to a very large effect size in therapy.

Clinical Decisions Making, Treatment Implementation, and Monitoring of Patient Progress. One of the methods that practitioners use to make decisions about clients and clinical work and to implement treatment is based on their intuition. While this is a valid way to make some decisions within interpersonal relationships, like all humans, practitioners can be highly biased. Thus, where possible, clinical intuition should be supported with clinical evidence based tools, such as monitoring the process and outcome of care.

> Clinical expertise also entails the monitoring of patient progress (and of changes in the patient's circumstances – e.g., job loss, major illness) that may suggest the need to adjust the treatment. (Lambert, Bergin, & Garfield, 2004)

As discussed later, practitioners can often miss these important makers in therapy, and as such, decisions regarding treatment implementation should be done using as many means as possible, including that of the client, standardised measures, and the practitioner's expertise and intuition.

Interpersonal Expertise. Interpersonal skills are fundamental to the therapeutic process and outcomes of care. Practitioners who can engage a wide range of diverse clients by building a therapeutic alliance, providing accurate empathy and who demonstrate advanced communication skills tend to be very effective. As we will see later, when examining the many variables that to contribute to effective psychotherapy, evidence based relationships impact greatly on the outcome of client care, and therapist vary greatly in their effectiveness. In a study, Anderson, Ogles, Patterson, Lambert, and Vermeersch (2009) demonstrated that facilitative interpersonal skills predict the outcome of therapists. Research also indicates that interpersonal facilitative skills help improve outcomes through allowing the practitioner to handle difficult interpersonal situations. More contemporary research in deliberate practice also demonstrates that practitioners can develop advanced interpersonal and communication skills through successive refinement and coaching that is generally not present in traditional training (Anderson, Perlman, McCarrick, & McClintock, 2019; Newman et al., 2022).

Continual Self-reflection and Acquisition of Skills. Clinical expertise also means taking a reflective position on our work: understanding our limitations, our scope of practice, our biases, our worldviews, and being able to reflect on these critically and reflect on how they impact our work. As we will see in a later chapter, practitioner's biases reach across all aspects of practice and in many cases, we are not aware of these limitations. Our biases can operate in the treatment strategies we use, the client type and issues we work with, how we conceptualise cases, and our overall clinical judgement. The APA suggest the following as methods to help develop clinical expertise in this area: research and theory; systematic clinical observation; hypothesis testing; self-reflection and feedback from other sources (e.g. supervisors, peers, client, other health professionals, the client's significant others, where appropriate); monitoring of client outcomes; and continuing education and other learning opportunities.

Appropriate Evaluation and Use of Research Evidence in Both Basic and Applied Psychological Science. An openness to using research is essential for the successful practitioner. A scientific enquiring mind is a hall mark of the scientist-practitioner. This means moving beyond theoretical orientations and seeking to integrate relevant research into one's practice at all levels. A grounding in research is essential for practitioners, as it allows them to draw inferences about different types of evidence within and across studies and the meaning this has for working with different people and populations. Understanding how different types of research evidence impacts on the generalisability of an intervention and the implication for the practitioner's given context is integral.

Understanding the Influence of Individual and Cultural Differences on Treatment. Clients will have differential needs based on their stage of development, age, gender, and other important demographics. Many factors influence the strategies practitioners will utilise, from age to certain cultural understandings of health and ill health. The needs of a developing adolescent are of course different to that of an adult entering the later stages of life, as are the worldviews and cognitive and emotional development needs. Likewise, the cultural context also needs to be considered, the explanatory model of health (Benish et al., 2011; Kleinman,

1980) of a Western client will likely be different to that from a client from an African country. Awareness of culture is discussed in a whole chapter later in this book, and is essential to positive outcomes (Huey, Tilley, Jones, & Smith, 2014).

Seeking Available Resources (E.g. Consultation, Adjunctive, or Alternative Services). Clients, their worries, and distress do not occur in a vacuum. Rather, clients' troubles can be impacted by, and in turn impact on, their biology, psychology, and social wellbeing. Practitioners must be able to draw on other resources, and where appropriate advocate, and make referrals to other services as necessary. For example, when a client is not making progress, medication may be warranted, or a physical illness which is making a client feel psychologically distressed may be helped by a referral to a doctor. In other cases, especially where culturally appropriate, referral to religious, spiritual, or traditional healers may be helpful. Practitioners should be mindful and aware of how their worldview can impact on making these referrals or seeking consultations with other types of support. Seeking consultation with a supervisor or coach is also important, we discuss how this can be used as a resource for quality assurance and developing further expertise in Part 3 of this book.

Having a Cogent Rationale for Clinical Strategies. In later chapters, I will speak on this topic further with reference to expectations and treatment credibility. However, briefly, practitioners must be able to confidently and with verbal consistency provide a rationale for the strategies and interventions that they will be using. The explanation provided to a client helps build the credibility of the provider. Assessment, case conceptualisation, and interventions all must be explained to the client with a compelling rationale, it must also be acceptable to the client, within their cultural context (APA, 2006).

Some rationales and strategies will be straight forward, such as explaining a behavioural protocol to a client experiencing depression that is based on research evidence. Other more complex conceptualisations may be based on the use of integrative or pluralistic (Norcross & Cooper, 2019) approaches that are seeking to explain the overall orientation of the practitioner, in the context of the client's wider reason for seeking help. Clinical expertise, thus, involves making sense of the client's presenting issues within the context of relevant theories and research, and articulating this to the client with as a way of explaining the client's difficulties, and treatment stategies.

Client Characteristics, Culture, and Preferences

The finial aspect of this tripartite model is for practitioners to be knowledgeable and efficient in working with client characteristics, culture, and preferences. Client characteristics occur across varied socioeconomic and cultural domains. Lifespan, age and the wider system that the client lives in all need to be considered. Other characteristics such as presenting problem, 'diagnoses', and motivation are also considered an important client characteristic. Culture is also essential, I have briefly discussed this above, and will do so in a later chapter. Multicultural considerations across race, ethnicity, socioeconomic status, disability, gender, and sex all play an important role in therapy. They influence how distress is understood, help seeking behaviours, and acceptable treatment approaches by the client (Benish et al., 2011; Huey et al., 2014). Likewise, considering preferences regarding the type, mode, modality, and style of therapy a client wishes to receive is important, and will be further discussed later in this book.

Conclusion

EBP is a complex concept and goes well beyond the idea of the treatment method, or empirically supported treatments. EBP as described in this chapter is based on a tripartite model consisting of best available research, clinical expertise, client characteristics, culture, and preferences. EBP speaks to the breadth and depth of the knowledge and expertise a practitioner must have. While EBP was designed as a guiding model for psychologists, most aspects of the model apply to those in allied professions where psychotherapeutic interventions are delivered. The model provides an excellent foundation for practitioners to think about how they approach their work, and the various types of evidence, research, and concepts that must be assimilated in therapy work. In the following chapter, I build on the idea of EBP by introducing the reader to non-specific components of therapy and the concept of the common factors as an alternative argument to the empirically supported treatments movement, but also as a complimentary necessity for effective therapy to occur.

References

American Psychological Association. (2002). Criteria for evaluating treatment guidelines. *American Psychologist*, *57*, 1052–1059.

American Psychological Association (APA). (2006). *Evidence based practice in psychology* (Vol. 61, No. 4, pp. 271–285). Washington, DC: American Psychological Association. 0003-066X/06/$12.00. doi:10.1037/0003-066X.61.4.271

American Psychological Association (APA). (2021). Professional practice guidelines for evidence-based psychological practice in health care. Retrieved from https://www.apa.org/about/policy/evidence-based-psychological-practice-health-care.pdf

Anderson, T., Ogles, B. M., Patterson, C. L., Lambert, M. J., & Vermeersch, D. A. (2009). Therapist effects: Facilitative interpersonal skills as a predictor of therapist success. *Journal of Clinical Psychology*, *65*, 755–768. https://doi.org/10.1002/jclp.20583

Anderson, T., Perlman, M. R., & McCarrick, S., McClintock, A. (2019). Modeling therapist responses with structured practice enhances facilitative interpersonal skills. *Journal of Clinical Psychology*, *76*(4), 659–675. https://doi.org/10.1002/jclp.22911

Beck, A. T., Epstein, N., Brown, G., & Steer, R. A. (1988). An inventory for measuring clinical anxiety: Psychometric properties. *Journal of Consulting and Clinical Psychology*, *56*(6), 893–897. https://doi.org/10.1037//0022-006x.56.6.893

Beck, A. T., Ward, C. H., Mendelson, M., Mock, J., & Erbaugh, J. (1961). An inventory for measuring depression. *Archives of General Psychiatry*, *4*, 561–571.

Benish, S. G., Quintana, S., & Wampold, B. E. (2011). Culturally adapted psychotherapy and the legitimacy of myth: A direct-comparison meta-analysis. *Journal of Counseling Psychology*, *58*(3), 279–289. https://doi.org/10.1037/a0023626

Brown, G. S. (J.), Simon, A., Cameron, J., & Minami, T. (2015). A collaborative outcome resource network (ACORN): Tools for increasing the value of psychotherapy. *Psychotherapy*, *52*(4), 412–421. https://doi.org/10.1037/pst0000033

Cooper, M., Norcross, J. C., Raymond-Barker, B., & Hogan, T. P. (2019). Psychotherapy preferences of laypersons and mental health professionals: Whose therapy is it? *Psychotherapy*, *56*(2), 205–216. https://doi.org/10.1037/pst0000226

Dragioti, E., Dimoliatis, I., & Evangelou, E. (2015). Disclosure of researcher allegiance in meta-analyses and randomised controlled trials of psychotherapy: A systematic appraisal. *BMJ Open*, *5*, e007206. doi:10.1136/bmjopen-2014-007206

Firth, N., Saxon, D., Stiles, W. B., & Barkham, M. (2019). Therapist and clinic effects in psychotherapy: A three-level model of outcome variability. *Journal of Consulting and Clinical Psychology*, *87*(4), 345–356. https://doi.org/10.1037/ccp0000388\

Huey, S. J., Jr, Tilley, J. L., Jones, E. O., & Smith, C. A. (2014). The contribution of cultural competence to evidence-based care for ethnically diverse populations. *Annual Review of Clinical Psychology*, *10*, 305–338. https://doi.org/10.1146/annurev-clinpsy-032813-153729

Johns, R. G., Barkham, M., Kellett, S., & Saxon, D. (2019). A systematic review of therapist effects: A critical narrative update and refinement to review. *Clinical Psychology Review*, *67*, 78–93. https://doi.org/10.1016/j.cpr.2018.08.004

Kleinman, A. (1980). *Patients and healers in the context of culture: An exploration of the borderland between anthropology, medicine, and psychiatry*. Berkeley, CA: University of California Press.

Lambert, M. J., Bergin, A. E., & Garfield, S. L. (2004). Introduction and historical overview. In M. J. Lambert (Ed.), *Bergin and Garfield's handbook of psychotherapy and behavior change* (5th ed., pp. 3–15). New York, NY: Wiley.

Munder, T., Flückiger, C., Gerger, H., Wampold, B. E., & Barth, J. (2012). Is the allegiance effect an epiphenomenon of true efficacy differences between treatments? A meta-analysis. *Journal of Counseling Psychology*, *59*(4), 631–637. https://doi.org/10.1037/a0029571

Newman, D. S., Villarreal, J. N., Gerrard, M. K., McIntire, H., Barrett, C. A., & Kaiser, L. T. (2022). Deliberate practice of consultation communication skills: A randomized controlled trial. *School Psychology*, *37*(3), 225–235. Advance online publication. https://doi.org/10.1037/spq0000494

Norcross, J. C. (Ed.). (2002). *Psychotherapy relationships that work: Therapist contributions and responsiveness to patients*. Oxford: Oxford University Press.

Rosenthal, R. (1990). How are we doing in soft psychology? *American Psychologist*, *45*, 775–777.

Sackett, D. L., Straus, S. E., Richardson, W. S., Rosenberg, W., & Haynes, R. B. (2000). *Evidence based medicine: How to practice and teach EBM* (2nd ed.). London: Churchill Livingstone.

Swift, J. K., Callahan, J. L., Cooper, M., & Parkin, S. R. (2018). The impact of accommodating client preference in psychotherapy: A meta-analysis. *Journal of Clinical Psychology*, *74*(11), 1924–1937. https://doi.org/10.1002/jclp.22680

Wampold, B. E., & Brown, G. S. (J.). (2005). Estimating variability in outcomes attributable to therapists: A naturalistic study of outcomes in managed care. *Journal of Consulting and Clinical Psychology*, *73*(5), 914–923. https://doi.org/10.1037/0022-006X.73.5.914

Wampold, B. E., & Imel, Z. E. (2015). *The great psychotherapy debate: The evidence for what makes psychotherapy work* (2nd ed.). New York, NY: Routledge.

Wampold, B. E., & Serlin, R. C. (2014). Meta-analytic methods to test relative efficacy. *Quality & Quantity: International Journal of Methodology*, *48*, 755–765. Retrieved from https://psycnet.apa.org/record/2014-04445-013. Accessed on March 3, 2020.

Chapter 3

The Common Factors in Therapy

Daryl Mahon

Abstract

In the previous chapters, we have explored some of the key debates around empirically supported treatments, and I have introduced the reader to the concept of evidence based practice as a tripartite model that speaks to a much wider understanding of therapy research and practice. In this chapter, I introduce the concept of the common factors and some of the research that supports the idea that in general all therapy approaches tend to be as effective as each other, indeed, a summary of this research going back as far as 1936 is highlighted. The common factor proposition rests on the premise that there are far more commonalities across diverse therapy methods, than differences, and that it is these trans-theoretical constructs that are responsible for the lion's share of outcomes. After briefly reviewing some of the literature, several common factor models are presented for the reader to consider.

Keywords: Common factors; dodo bird; equivalence; contextual model; psychotherapy research; relative effects

Chapter Learning Outcomes

(1) Understand the research supporting the common factor proposition.
(2) Examine a range of common factor models.

Introduction

> Everybody has won, and all must have prizes.

It is quite astonishing to think that it was in 1936 that Saul Rosenzweig wrote the classic, but still not well known paper, *Some Implicit Common Factors in Diverse*

Evidence Based Counselling & Psychotherapy for the 21st Century Practitioner, 27–36

Published under exclusive licence by Emerald Publishing Limited
doi:10.1108/978-1-80455-732-720231003

Methods of Psychotherapy. The paper is the first known articulation of the common factor proposition in psychotherapy. As this chapter will set out, the common factors refer to different processes that occur across all psychotherapies regardless of the theoretical modality that is being delivered. That is, common factors are said to be trans-theoretical methods and processes involved in the effective delivery of psychotherapy and resulting outcomes, they are non-specific to any one theory (Ahn & Wampold, 2001; Cuijpers, Reijnders, & Huibers, 2019; Duncan, Hubble, & Miller, 2010; Frank, 1961; Luborsky, Singer, & Luborsky, 1975; Rosenzweig, 1936; Wampold & Imel, 2008). In comparison, you will remember from Chapter 1 when we discussed the role of empirically supported treatments which are said to have remedial ingredients that are specific and necessary to treat specific 'disorders' (Chambless & Hollon, 1998) and based on a medical model of psychopathology (Duncan, 2002).

Interestingly, Rosenzweig (1936) suggested that the common factors are so embedded in psychotherapies that there would be little to no difference found in the effectiveness of diverse approaches. Drawing on the quote above, taken from Lewis Carroll's *Alice in Wonderland* story, Rosenzweig made the comparison from the dodo bird who was asked to judge a race, and proclaimed, 'Everybody has won, and all must have prizes'. It would be many years before innovations in empirical research were powerful enough to test this postulate, and what follows is a short summary of the trajectory this research has taken.

Support for the Dodo Verdict

The first comparative study to confirm Rosenzweig's (1936) hypotheses was a study carried out by Luborsky, Singer, and Luborsky (1975). Having examined 100 comparative studies, the authors concluded that there was little to no meaningful difference between studies. Luborsky also suggested that 'Everybody has won, and all must have prizes.' Around this time, the authors of the study, and other researchers in the field began to refer to this phenomena as the Dodo Bird Verdict. Luborsky's study was replicated by Smith, Glass, and Miller (1980), using a much larger sample of 475 studies. In a review of 17 meta-analyses examining the Dodo Verdict, Luborsky et al. (2002, p. 8) concluded that:

> Rosenzweig's clinically-based hypothesis of 1936 has held up – the outcomes of quantitative comparisons of different active treatments with each other, because of their similar major components, are likely to show mostly 'small' and nonsignificant differences from each other.

Some might consider this research old and outdated, or suggest that more powerful research methods are now available and able to capture more nuanced treatment effects. However, a review of more recent research, including meta-analyses across various constructs leads us to similar conclusions. For example, in substance use (Imel, Wampold, Miller, & Fleming, 2008) meta-analysis found that when researcher allegiance was controlled for, outcomes tended to be equivalent across treatment approaches, other research in the substance use space came to findings of the same nature (Project Match Research Group, 1998). When examining eating disorders, Spielmans et al.'s (2013) meta-analysis found no difference between bona fide approaches, nor was there any difference between approaches intended to be therapeutic in a meta-analysis for treatment of youth anxiety and depression (Miller, Wampold, & Varhely, 2008).

The area of trauma and post-traumatic stress disorder is increasingly proliferating the literature with 'new' models of treatment being developed regularly. However, as Benish et al. (2008) demonstrated in their meta-analysis, there was no difference between comparative treatments in their study. In their meta-analysis, Hoogsteder, Ten Thije, Schippers, and Stams (2022) comparing trauma-focussed treatments, whereas both trauma-focussed cognitive behavioural therapy (TF-CBT) and eye movement and desensitisation reprocessing (EMDR) were more effective than no treatment; they were not more effective than treatment as usual. The only meta-analysis conducted into the use of EMDR in trauma found that when bias was controlled for, that all approaches in the study tended to be equally effective (Cuijpers, Veen, Sijbrandij, Yoder, & Cristea, 2020).

Strong evidence for the common factor postulate can be inferred through dismantling studies, that is, studies that remove the proposed specific ingredient of change. Dismantling studies have demonstrated that when specific ingredients are removed from trauma-focussed therapies, the remaining treatment component has demonstrated equivalence with the full treatment, including removing the eye movements in EMDR treatment. The same has been found in CBT when the behavioural component is removed (Bell, Marcus, & Goodlad, 2013; Cahill, Carrigan, & Frueh, 1999). Strong evidence exists that demonstrates on the whole the treatment method while needed of course, in general does not matter which approach is used, and any differences tend to be small, not clinically meaningful, or statistically significant. However, there have been some exceptions to this (Cuijpers et al., 2019), but these results are often refuted on methodological grounds. As such, learning to leverage big impactful common factors may be a more fruitful approach taken to improve effectiveness.

Common Factor Models

While the previous research attests to the fact that there is little to no meaningful difference between approaches intended to be therapeutic (bona fide), the question then becomes what are these common factors that authors speak of. Rosenzweig (1936) was the first to articulate this presupposition, and others followed in his footsteps. Carl Rogers (1957) published his core condition which he thought to be necessary and sufficient, while Frank (1961) was one of the next authors to write about the common factors across therapies. Frank identified four factors that he viewed as common across diverse approaches:

(1) An emotionally charged, confiding relationship with a helping person.
(2) A healing setting.

(3) A rationale, conceptual scheme, or myth that provides a plausible explanation for the client's symptoms and prescribe a ritual or procedure for resolving them.
(4) A ritual or procedure that requires the active participation of both client and therapist and that is believed by both to be the means of restoring the client's health.

Orlinsky and Howard (1986) proposed five process variables that are active in any psychotherapy: the therapeutic contract, therapeutic interventions, the therapeutic bond between therapist and client, the client's and therapist's states of self-relatedness, and therapeutic realisation. However, the first empirical study to distil common factors may be traced back to Grencavage and Norcross (1990). After reviewing the literature of 50 articles they concluded that:

> Analyses revealed that 41% of proposed commonalities were change processes; by contrast, only 6% of articulated commonalities were client characteristics. The most consensual commonalities across categories were development of a therapeutic alliance, opportunity for catharsis, acquisition and practice of new behaviours, and clients' positive expectancies.

As we can see there is already commonalities in the different common factor models. Similarly, Lambert (1992) provided a summary of the literature and identified what he considered to be the percentage that certain common factors contributed to change.

(1) Extra-therapeutic change (40%), those factors that are qualities of the client or qualities of his or her environment.
(2) Common factors (30%) that are found in a variety of therapy approaches, such as empathy and the therapeutic relationship.
(3) Expectancy (15%), the portion of improvement that results from the client's expectation of help or belief in the rationale or effectiveness of therapy.
(4) Techniques (15%), those factors unique to specific therapies and tailored to treatment of specific problems.

The work of Lambert led to researchers Duncan, Hubble, and Miller (2010, *The Heart and Soul of Change*) to set out a common factor model that depicts the various common factors with the variance in change attributable to each. I discuss these factors below. One of the critical points that many who discuss the common factors miss is that this is not a model that you bring together in an integrative manner. No, these are components of all therapies, while feedback is the most recent addition, and not all practitioners use it, or are aware of it for that matter, the common factors exist in all therapies, however, some practitioners may be more proficient at leveraging them, and it is this difference that I propose as accounting for the vast difference between diverse practitioner's ability to effect change.

Client/Life Factors

Like Lambert before them who suggested extra-therapeutic factors, this model refers to client/life factors and unexplained variance. Client factors are those things that a client brings to therapy, their existing or non-existent psychological, social, and physical capital. For example, social connections and community, strong ego strength, financial capital, and employment. As such, client/life factors are not influenced by the therapist and provide individuals with resources that help alleviate distress, or indeed mean a client will have better resources available to manage life. For example, a client who is experiencing a sense of loss and emotional distress after breaking up with a partner suddenly reunites, or the client who is feeling depressed after losing their employment suddenly finds a new employment opportunity. These are issues outside the therapist's ability to effect, and are thus, extra-therapeutic/life factors. In this model, Duncan (2014) suggests a variance of up to 86% of change is accounted for by client/life factors and unexplained variances. To draw a comparison, in medicine, medical care only accounts for approximately 10-20% of modifiable contributors to healthy outcomes, with 80-90% coming from what is termed social determinants of health, such as health-related behaviors, socioeconomic factors, and environmental factors. The social determinants of health is medicines equivalent to extra-therapeutic factors.

Therapeutic Alliance

The therapeutic alliance is perhaps the strongest predictor of change and whether therapy is going to be successful. The alliance is conceptualised based on the work of Bordin (1976) and consists of the bond between the practitioner and the client, the extent of the agreement on the goals and the tasks of therapy. My colleagues Dr Jeb Brown, Ashely Simon, and I have recently illustrated the power of the alliance in therapy which I will discuss in a subsequent chapter.

Feedback Effects

The use of feedback is a new addition to the common factor research, and I discuss it later on as a powerful variable. Feedback effects refer to the use of instruments to solicit feedback on the process and outcome of care, and to use the resulting information to adapt the treatment experience based on the client's wishes, needs, and preferences in real time. Feedback/routine monitoring as we seen earlier is another recommendation from the APA and is incorporated into evidence based practice (EBP).

Model/Technique Specific Effects

The specific effects are those ingredients that a modality puts forward as the specific change mechanism, the protocols that make them different from another. As is illustrated from the chart, and indeed the research, any differences found are small and not meaningful. According to Wampold and Imel, specific effects of therapies account for about between 0-2% of the outcomes.

Model/Technique General Effects

The general effects are with regard to the delivery of the treatment, and are based on the therapist's allegiance to their methods, their ability to explain to clients presenting problems, and described a set of rituals or techniques that can alleviate the client's distress based on the explanation of the presenting problems. This helps build expectancy, instil hope, or what we can also refer to as the placebo effect.

Therapist Effects

Therapist's effects refer to the difference between practitioners and their ability to bring about positive outcomes in the lives of their clients. Critically, therapist's effects have little to do with the modality of therapy. Research suggests that there is substantial difference between therapists. Therapist effects are still being researched and the field is attempting to understand how and why there can be so much differences, especially if it is the treatment method that is accounting for change as suggested by the empirically supported treatment position.

Contextual Common Factors

The most modern and well-developed common factors model is perhaps the contextual model by Wampold (2015). This model is proposed as an alternative to the medical model or empirically supported treatments in which therapies are supposed to work through specific ingredients that are 'purportedly beneficial for particular disorders due to remediation of an identifiable deficit' (Wampold, 2015, p. 270). In the contextual model, a client and a therapist must first create a basic bond with each other as a foundation before work begins. After the establishment of this bond, therapy is argued to work through three pathways.

The first pathway is the real relationship, which Gelso (2014, p. 119) suggests as 'the personal relationship between therapist and patient marked by the extent to which each is genuine with the other and perceives/experiences the other in ways that befit the other'. This relationship provides the client with a connection to a caring therapist who wishes to help. This dynamic is assumed to be healing, especially for clients who encounter difficulties in social relationships. Pathway two is through a client's hope and expectancy built by the therapist. Therapies need to provide an explanation for how the client developed mental health difficulties and pathways to healing. The therapy and therapist provide clients with a means to cope with or solve their problems, they instil hope, and provide tasks that can help the client deal with, manage, and resolve the issues that they find distressing.

The final pathway consists of the specific/active ingredients of therapies. These specific ingredients create expectations in our clients and activate pathway two and produce some salubrious actions (Wampold, 2015). These actions and tasks will be different depending on the therapy. For example, they may help improve the clients' social relationships (interpersonal psychotherapy), or in adopting a more helpful ways of thinking (cognitive therapy), or help a client become more self-aware and have insight into their problems (psychodynamic therapy). An important point is that these methods do not work like a medicine. A strong therapeutic alliance is essential for both the second and third paths to be activated. As Cuijpers et al. (2019, p. 2010) inform us:

> It is not assumed that these specific ingredients exert a direct effect through the medical model by repairing an apparent deficit, but rather that, in general, they stimulate healthy actions that are beneficial to clients.

Impact of Contextual Common Factors

Not only did Wampold (2015) provide us with a common factor model, but he also provided a description of the impact of the common factor and specific factor variables on the therapy process by identifying their effect size on the therapy outcome. In the final chapter, I provide a similar outline that can be used for practitioner development. My colleague Jeb discusses effect size in his technology chapter later on, but to give you an idea as to their meaning as I refer to effect size lots in the subsequent chapters. To understand the importance of effects, Cohen classified a *d* of 0.2 as small, 0.5 as medium, and 0.8 as large.

As illustrated in the various common factor models discussed in this chapter, many of the models discuss similar ideas and concepts, and there is a great deal of consistency across models. However, it is important to point out that the evidence derived for the common factors is largely correlational, and as such, whether change happens because of these factors is still under scrutiny in the same way that specific ingredients cannot be conclusively proven to be the cause of change.

To sum up, I draw on a paper in The Annual Review of Clinical Psychology. Cuijpers et al. (2019) provide the following summary regarding the state of the research base for specific and non-specific psychotherapy processes and outcomes:

(1) Although hundreds of randomised controlled trials have shown that psychotherapies are effective in treating mental health difficulties, it is not known how they work.
(2) Therapies may work through techniques that are specific to each therapy, through factors that all therapies have in common, or through a combination of the two.
(3) The discussion about whether therapies work through common or specific mechanisms has been going on for several decades, but it has not been resolved because it is not known how therapies work.
(4) Meta-analyses of comparative outcome studies do not all point to comparable effects for different therapies and because alternative explanations are possible for comparable effects, it is not known whether all therapies do, in fact, have comparable effects.
(5) Component studies (in which one component is removed from or added to a therapy and this is compared with the complete therapy) are also inconclusive, regardless of whether specific components are partly responsible for the effects of therapies.

(6) There is no straightforward method for examining how therapies work, and most research on specific and common factors has been conducted using correlational studies; there has been little research on temporal associations, dose–response relationships, supportive theoretical frameworks, and laboratory studies.
(7) Although hundreds of correlational studies have been conducted during the past decades, little progress has been made in understanding the mechanisms of change of therapies: It is as if we have been in a pilot phase of research for five decades.

Conclusion

It has been almost 90 years since the seminal paper written by Saul Rosenzweig, and in many ways, not much has changed, other than that there is substantially more modalities for practitioners to choose from today then there were in the period when Saul was writing about therapy. However, over these last 90 years the research has remained largely consistent, in that generally therapies are found to be equivalent on the whole, with any differences often being non-significant and not clinically meaningful. This is not to say that anything goes, or that at different times or with different clients some therapies don't perform better, because they can, and sometimes do. Yet, when this does occur we can often find some of the reasons for this in the common factors and the practitioner as opposed to the specific therapy or ingredient. In the subsequent chapters, I will provide an overview of the variables that are correlated with positive outcomes in therapy and how these key areas impact outcomes across therapies in general. However, we must also realise that the treatment method is important, or in the words of Frank & Frank, (1991, p. xv):

> My position is not that technique is irrelevant to outcome. Rather, I maintain that … the success of all techniques depends on the patient's sense of alliance with an actual or symbolic healer. This position implies that ideally therapists should select for each patient the therapy that accords, or can be brought to accord, with the patient's personal characteristics and view of the problem.

References

Ahn, H.-n., & Wampold, B. E. (2001). Where oh where are the specific ingredients? A meta-analysis of component studies in counseling and psychotherapy. *Journal of Counseling Psychology*, *48*(3), 251–257. https://doi.org/10.1037/0022-0167.48.3.25

Bell, E. C., Marcus, D. K., & Goodlad, J. K. (2013). Are the parts as good as the whole? A meta-analysis of component treatment studies. *Journal of Consulting and Clinical Psychology*, *81*, 722–736.

Benish, S. G., Imel, Z. E., & Wampold, B. E. (2008). The relative efficacy of bona fide psychotherapies for treating post-traumatic stress disorder: A meta-analysis of direct comparisons. *Clinical Psychology Review*, *28*(5), 746–758. https://doi.org/10.1016/j.cpr.2007.10.005

Bordin, E. S. (1979). The generalizability of the psychoanalytic concept of the working alliance. *Psychotherapy: Theory, Research & Practice*, *16*(3), 252–260. https://doi.org/10.1037/h0085885

Cahill, S. P., Carrigan, M. H., & Frueh, B. C. (1999). Does EMDR work? And if so, why? A critical review of controlled outcome and dismantling research. *Journal of Anxiety Disorders*, *13*, 5–33.

Chambless, D. L., & Hollon, S. D. (1998). Defining empirically supported therapies. *Journal of Consulting and Clinical Psychology*, *66*, 7–18. Retrieved from https://www.ncbi.nlm.nih.gov/pubmed. Accessed on September 7, 2019.

Cuijpers, P., Reijnders, M., & Huibers, J. H. (2019). The role of the common factors in psychotherapy outcomes. *Annual Review of Clinical Psychology*, *15*, 207–231. https://www.annualreviews.org/doi/full/10.1146/annurev-clinpsy-050718-095424

Cuijpers, P., Veen, S., Sijbrandij, M., Yoder, W., & Cristea, I. A. (2020). Eye movement desensitization and reprocessing for mental health problems: A systematic review and meta-analysis. *Cognitive Behaviour Therapy*, *49*(3), 165–180. https://doi.org/10.1080/16506073.2019.1703801

Duncan, B. L. (2002). The legacy of Saul Rosenzweig: The profundity of the dodo bird. *Journal of Psychotherapy Integration*, *12*(1), 32–57. https://doi.org/10.1037/1053-0479.12.1.32

Duncan, B. L. (2014). *On becoming a better therapist* (2nd ed.). Washington, DC: American Psychological Association.

Duncan, B. L., Miller, S. D., Wampold, B. E., & Hubble, M. A. (Eds.). (2010). (2nd ed.). Washington, DC: American Psychological Association. https://doi.org/10.1037/12075-000

Frank, J. (1961). *Persuasion and healing: A comparative study of psychotherapy*. London: Johns Hopkins University Press.

Frank, J. D., & Frank, J. B. (1991). *Persuasion and healing: A comparative study of psychotherapy* (3rd ed.). Baltimore, MD: Johns Hopkins University Press.

Gelso C. (2014). A tripartite model of the therapeutic relationship: Theory, research, and practice. Psychotherapy research. *Journal of the Society for Psychotherapy Research*, *24*(2), 117–131. https://doi.org/10.1080/10503307.2013.845920

Grencavage, L. M., & Norcross, J. C. (1990). Where are the commonalities among the therapeutic common factors? *Professional Psychology: Research and Practice*, *21*(5), 372–378. https://doi.org/10.1037/0735-7028.21.5.372

Hoogsteder, L. M., Ten Thije, L., Schippers, E. E., & Stams, G. (2022). A meta-analysis of the effectiveness of EMDR and TF-CBT in reducing trauma symptoms and externalizing behavior problems in adolescents. *International Journal of Offender Therapy and Comparative Criminology*, *66*(6–7), 735–757. https://doi.org/10.1177/0306624X211010290

Imel, Z. E., Wampold, B. E., Miller, S. D., & Fleming, R. R. (2008). Distinctions without a difference: Direct comparisons of psychotherapies for alcohol use disorders. *Psychology of Addictive Behaviors: Journal of the Society of Psychologists in Addictive Behaviors*, *22*(4), 533–543. https://doi.org/10.1037/a0013171

Lambert, M. J (1992). Psychotherapy outcome research: Implications for integrative and eclectic therapists. In J. C. Norcross & M. R. Goldfried (Eds.), *Handbook of psychotherapy integration* (1st ed., pp. 94–129), New York, NY: Basic Books.

Luborsky, L., Rosenthal, R., Diguer, L., Andrusyna, T. P., Berman, J. S., Levitt, J. T., Seligman, D. A., & Krause, E. D. (2002). The dodo bird verdict is alive and well – Mostly. *Clinical Psychology: Science and Practice*, *9*(1), 2–12. https://doi.org/10.1093/clipsy.9.1.2

Luborsky, L., Singer, B., & Luborsky, L. (1975). Comparative studies of psychotherapies: Is it true that "everyone has won and all must have prizes"? *Archives of General Psychiatry*, *32*(8), 995–1008. https://doi.org/10.1001/archpsyc.1975.01760260059004

Miller, S., Wampold, B., & Varhely, K. (2008). Direct comparisons of treatment modalities for youth disorders: A meta-analysis. *Psychotherapy research: journal of the Society for Psychotherapy Research*, *18*(1), 5–14. https://doi.org/10.1080/10503300701472131

Orlinsky, D. E., & Howard, K. I. (1986). The psychological interior of psychotherapy: Explorations with the therapy session reports. In L. S. Greenberg & W. M. Pinsof (Eds.), *The psychotherapeutic process: A research handbook* (pp. 477–501). New York, NY: Guilford Press.

Project Match Research Group. (1998). Matching patients with alcohol disorders to treatments: Clinical implications from Project MATCH. *Journal of Mental Health*, *7*(6), 589–602. doi:10.1080/09638239817743

Rogers, C. R. (1957). The necessary and sufficient conditions of therapeutic personality change. *Journal of Consulting Psychology*, *21*(2), 95–103. https://doi.org/10.1037/h0045357

Rosenzweig, S. l. (1936). Some implicit common factors in diverse methods of psychotherapy. *American Journal of Orthopsychiatry*, *6*(3), 412–415. Retrieved from https://onlinelibrary.wiley.com/doi/abs/10.1111/j.1939-0025.1936.tb05248. Accessed on September 8.

Smith, M. L., Glass, G. V., & Miller, T. I. (1980). *The benefits of psychotherapy*. Baltimore, MD: John Hopkins University Press.

Spielmans, G. I., Benish, S. G., Marin, C., Bowman, W. M., Menster, M., & Wheeler, A. J. (2013). Specificity of psychological treatments for bulimia nervosa and binge eating disorder? A meta-analysis of direct comparisons. *Clinical Psychology Review*, *33*(3), 460–469. https://doi.org/10.1016/j.cpr.2013.01.008

Wampold, B. E. (2015). How important are the common factors in psychotherapy? An update. *World Psychiatry: Official Journal of the World Psychiatric Association (WPA)*, *14*(3), 270–277. https://doi.org/10.1002/wps.20238

Wampold, B. E., & Imel, Z. E. (2015). *The great psychotherapy debate: The evidence for what makes psychotherapy work* (2nd ed.). New York, NY: Routledge.

Part 2

Evidence Based Relationships & Responsiveness

Chapter 4

Evidence Based Relationships 1: Therapeutic Alliance, Goals and Collaboration, Alliance Rupture–Repair, and Feedback-informed Care

Daryl Mahon

Abstract

In the previous chapter, I introduced the reader to the ideas and research of the common factors. The common factors are varied and have demonstrated to have small to large effect sizes depending on what variable is being examined. In this chapter, I categorise four more evidence based relationship variables which tend to be more task orientated and aligned to the therapeutic alliance. Indeed, the therapeutic alliance, goals and collaboration, alliance rupture–repair, and feedback-informed care are four trans-theoretical factors that can contribute greatly to outcomes. At the same time, when poorly established they can and do impact negatively on client outcomes. This is not an exhaustive overview of the literature, rather each variable is briefly discussed, the evidence supporting the effectiveness is highlighted, and Top Tips are provided to assist the development of the practitioner.

Keywords: Therapeutic alliance; alliance rupture–repair; goals; collaboration; feedback-informed treatment; psychotherapy outcomes

Chapter Learning Outcomes

(1) Examine four evidence based relationship variables.
(2) Appreciate the interconnectedness and application of these variables.

Evidence Based Counselling & Psychotherapy for the 21st Century Practitioner, 39–51

Published under exclusive licence by Emerald Publishing Limited
doi:10.1108/978-1-80455-732-720231004

Introduction

Successful therapy occurs when there is an agreement between the practitioner and client with regard to the nature of the problem, the goals of therapy, and how these goals will be worked towards within a cultivated relational bond, that is, the therapeutic alliance. When these aspects of the alliance and goal attainment are in place, the treatment delivered produces better outcomes. However, alignment is something to be worked on continuously throughout the therapy process. Thus, practitioners must not only cultivate the alliance, but identify ruptures when they occur, and repair these as they relate to the bond between them and client, the extent of goal collaboration, and the individual tasks to be worked on. This is not always easy to do or achieve, yet it is imperative that it be done, outcomes depend on it. Using client feedback is another way alliances can be cultivated, ruptures can be identified, and goals and outcomes can be monitored. This is attained by listening to the client's experience of the process (alliance) and outcome (goals) of care on a regular basis. This chapter situates these evidence based relationship factors in the literature with regard to outcomes.

Goals Consensus and Collaboration

Goal consensus and goal attainment are a basic function of therapy through which clients bring about the type of change that they desire, whatever the presenting problem may be. As such, whether a client is engaged in classical analysis or cognitive behavioural therapy, goals will be part of the therapeutic process and are therefore a pan-theoretical construct across theories (Bordin, 1979). Goals are an essential part of the process from early in treatment, and must be negotiated and worked on between the client and the practitioner through a collaborative dialogue for the duration of therapy. Consequently, goal consensus is an important part of the contract between practitioner and client, and it is closely linked to and overlaps with the therapeutic alliance (discussed below). Collaboration is the process that informs the agreement between both parties of how the goals will be worked on (Tryon, Birch, & Verkuilen, 2018). A working definition of goal consensus is taken from Tryon and Winograd (2011), and consists of the following:

1. Client–practitioner agreement on and commitment to goals and how they will be achieved.
2. Client–practitioner agreement on the presenting problem.
3. The extent to which goals are articulated, discussed, and clearly defined.

In comparison, collaboration is a dynamic process that involves the active working on goals to achieve the desired outcomes, or as Kazantzis and Kellis (2012, p. 133) describe it:

> Collaboration between a psychotherapist and a patient occurs at the intersection of the therapeutic relationship and treatment method. Many methods contribute to collaboration, which is then experienced as a respectful, mutual, cooperative relationship.

As we can see this definition again fits the idea of collaboration being a pan-theoretical construct that is used by all practitioners and a part of all therapies. Similarly, as with the definition of goal consensus mentioned previously, a definition of collaboration is provided by Tryon and Winograd (2001, p. 157) as 'the mutual involvement of psychotherapist and patient in a helping relationship'. Thus, collaboration and goals consensus are part of the practitioner being responsive to the client's needs.

Impact of Goal Consensus and Collaboration on Outcomes

Three previous meta-analytic reviews can help us understand the relationships between goal consensus, collaboration, and outcomes. Tryon and Winograd (2001) included 25 studies in their goal consensus arm and found that 68% had a positive outcome between consensus and outcome. For collaboration–outcome relationship 89% of 24 studies demonstrated a positive outcome. In a 2011 meta-analysis, the same authors reported medium effect sizes for goal consensus on outcomes (15 studies) and a medium effect size for collaboration on outcomes (19 studies). The most recent meta-analysis (Tryon et al., 2018) reported that the goal consensus–outcome correlation for 54 studies was a medium effect size of d=0.49. The collaboration–outcome association for 53 studies also reported a medium effect size of d=0.61. It proves difficult to establish any moderators of these relationships other than that of homework, which also shows a relationship with consensus and outcome.

The research does not provide us with any implications for diversity as much of the included studies did not report on these characteristics.

Top Tips

1. Therapeutic work should only begin after goals consensus has been reached and the means to achieving these goals has been established.
2. Listen to client's explicit and implicit goals, seek their input, and don't push your own agenda. Being on the same page is integral. Seek feedback from the client throughout treatment to maintain alignment with goals and progress.
3. Develop collaborative homework assignments and encourage the client's engagement in homework completion. Start off with small tasks before moving onto more complex goals.
4. Solicit feedback from clients on their progress, functioning, and experience of care. Also, provide clients with regular feedback on their progress.
5. Use client feedback to modify your treatment approach, be conscious of ethical mandates to adapt a new stance should it be indicated based on client feedback .
6. Discuss clients' goals as positively valanced (what they want to achieve as opposed to what they want to stop doing or give up).

Therapeutic Alliance

The origins of the therapeutic alliance can be traced back to psychodynamic thinking, and is now firmly established as a common factor variable across theoretical modalities. Indeed, it has extended its reach beyond psychotherapy and into related allied health fields such as social work, nursing, psychiatry, medicine, and rehabilitation (Flückiger, Del Re, Wampold, & Horvath, 2018). There has been a number of authors proposing definitions of the alliance in the extant literature (Greenson, 1965; Zetzel, 1956). However, the one often used is based on a trans-theoretical conceptualisation put forward by Bordin (1976), who defined the alliance as the extent of the agreement on the therapeutic goals, consensus on the tasks that make up therapy, and a bond between the client and the practitioner. Indeed, it was Bordin who suggested that different therapies would place different demands on the relationship, thus the 'profile' of the ideal working alliance would differ across orientations (Flückiger et al., 2018). As we can see in these descriptions, the previous factors of goal consensus and collaboration are closely related.

Impact of Alliance on Outcomes

The alliance is one of the most studied variables in the psychotherapy literature (Norcross & Lambert, 2019) with well over 1,000 studies demonstrating its effectiveness as a common factor. In addition to this, the alliance is a robust predictor of client outcome (Flückiger et al., 2018, 2020; Wampold & Imel, 2015) and it contributes more to client outcomes than the treatment method (Wampold & Imel, 2015).

In addition, therapists who can build an alliance with a wider range of clients tend to have better outcomes (Baldwin, Wampold, & Imel, 2007). Moreover, the practitioner's contribution to the alliance is thought to be more important than the client's (Del Re, Flückiger, Horvath, Symonds, & Wampold, 2012).

There has been about eight meta-analyses conducted that have examined the alliance–outcome correlation since 1991, with surprisingly similar findings even with advanced methodologies that can detect more nuances in later years. Early alliance predicts approximately 5% of the variance in treatment outcomes (Flückiger et al., 2018). In their meta-analysis with a dataset of 5,350, Flückiger et al. (2020) found improvements in alliance scores in one session are associated with reductions in symptoms in subsequent sessions. 'Findings provide reciprocally related to one other, often resulting in a positive upward spiral of higher alliance/lower symptoms that predicted higher alliances/lower symptoms in the subsequent sessions'.

The most recent meta-analysis (Flückiger et al., 2018) syntheses 295 studies with 30,000 participants. Findings are consistent with the previous studies with a moderate effect size of d=0.579, which indicates that the alliance–outcome relationship contributes about 8% to the variability in outcome. The study provides some interesting research related to possible moderators of the alliance–outcome correlations. This relation remains consistent across assessor perspectives, alliance and outcome measures, treatment approaches, client characteristics, and countries. While there was no difference in findings based on presenting issues (personality disorder, anxiety, etc.), substance use seems to be the one factor that the outcome correlation is moderated by, with smaller effect sizes in those clients presenting with substance use issues. Again, diversity factors were not captured in this large study, although other research projects on multicultural orientation suggest that the alliance is mediated by cultural humility.

Top Tips

1. Establish the alliance early on in therapy, by creating a warm relational bond and a collaborative attachment with the client.
2. Practitioners should develop the goals and tasks in a collaborative manner early on in therapy.
3. Practitioners should be responsive and address ruptures in the alliance at the point they occur.
4. Being responsive by assessing and monitoring the alliance on an ongoing basis can reduce drop-out and improve outcomes.
5. Mirror the clients motivational level and stage of stage early on.
6. The alliance is based on negotiation, this extends to the goals and tasks also.
7. Don't assume that an early strong alliance means later alliance will also be strong, practitioners must work throughout therapy to cultivate the alliance.

Alliance Rupture–Repair

As outlined above, the strength of the evidence for the therapeutic alliance being a predictor of psychotherapy outcome is impressive. Thus, it seems reasonable that practitioners should maintain and tend to the alliance in order to influence outcomes. However, as with all human relationship (which the alliance reflects), ruptures occur for various reasons.

Eubanks, Muran, and Safran (2018, p. 508) define an alliance rupture as

> a deterioration in the therapeutic alliance, manifested by a disagreement between the patient and therapist on treatment goals, a lack of collaboration on therapeutic tasks, or a strain in their emotional bond.

While some therapies will consider the alliance as the centre focus of the work, other modalities see it as less important. However regardless of the importance that the alliance is considered to have by different orientations it is important for the client and the strongest predictor of outcomes.

The term rupture may conjure up visions of heated disagreements and emotive interactions. However, although this may occur in a small minority of cases, alliance ruptures are often much more nuanced, and many may even go unnoticed, as described by Eubanks et al. (2018, p. 509), 'Although the term rupture may connote a dramatic breakdown in the therapeutic relationship, many studies of alliance ruptures also regard subtle tensions and minor misattunements as markers of ruptures'. Given how nuanced and subtle these stresses on the alliance can be, it is imperative that the practitioner can identify and repair such ruptures as soon as possible. Yet, to do this, the practitioner must first have a way to conceptualise a rupture and a lens to view the alliance rupture through. Alliance ruptures tend to be operationalised in two ways: withdrawal rupture and confrontational rupture (Safran & Muran, 2000).

Withdrawal ruptures involve the client moving away from the practitioner and the therapeutic process, for example, by avoiding the practitioner's engagement or by hiding his or her dissatisfaction with therapy or the practitioner. In comparison, confrontation ruptures occur when the client moves towards the practitioner by expressing hostilities such as anger or unhappiness with the practitioner or treatment process, or by trying to exert pressure or control the practitioner (Eubanks et al., 2018). Ruptures are generally deemed to be mended when the practitioner and client are back working collaboratively, and the bond is re-established (Eubanks-Carter, 2010). Practitioners will find the following withdrawal and confrontational rupture markers (Table 4) as a helpful lens to identify, view, and be responsive to ruptures, however, it is not an exhaustive list. It is not only identifying ruptures that can be difficult, but practitioners may also find it difficult to manage their feelings related to ruptures. For example, Eubanks, Sergi, and Muran (2021, p. 86) postulate that 'working with ruptures can evoke feelings in the therapist that are difficult to tolerate; experiences such as confusion, incompetence, guilt, and irritation are not uncommon'.

Table 4. Types of Alliance Ruptures.

Withdrawal Rupture Markers	**Confrontational Rupture Markers**
Denial	Complaints/concerns about the therapist
Minimal response	Client rejects therapist intervention
Abstract communication	Complaints/concerns about the activities of therapy
Avoidant storytelling and/or shifting topic	Complaints/concerns about the parameters of therapy
Deferential and appeasing	Complaints/concerns about progress in therapy
Content/affect split	Client defends self against therapist
Self-criticism and/or hopelessness	Efforts to control/pressure therapist

Impact of Alliance Rupture–Repair on Outcome

In the previous meta-analysis, Safran, Muran, and Eubanks-Carter (2011) illustrated the rupture–repair strategies in session, and rupture–repair training were moderately related to therapy outcomes. The most recent meta-analysis addressed the same two alliance rupture–repair training questions with a larger sample. In 11 studies with 1,314 participants, Eubanks et al. (2018) found a moderate effect size of d=0.62 between rupture–repair and client outcome. When exploring possible moderators of this outcome, the researchers examined whether clients' characteristics such as personality disorder, experience of therapist (trainee vs experienced), or treatment modality (psychodynamic vs cognitive behavioural therapy (CBT)) played a part in these findings, there was no findings to support any of these areas as moderators. However, one moderator did almost approach statistical significance, studies that measured the alliance later in care tended to have a stronger outcome correlation than those that measured early in care.

This moderator is reflective of findings from two studies by my colleagues and myself. Dr Jeb Brown, Ashley Simon, and I analysed the relationship between the alliance and outcome of therapy in the first five sessions (Mahon, Brown, & Simon, 2021a) and the alliance–outcome correlation for 5–20 sessions (Mahon, Brown, & Simon, 2021b). There are two main findings from these studies that support this moderator and further extend our knowledge on the importance of rupture–repair and client outcomes. The sample size in these studies was much larger, with 41,171 participants. The first finding of interest supports the tentative conclusions drawn in the Eubanks et al.'s (2018) study, average alliance scores early in treatment were not predictive of change at later sessions. Only the average alliance scores for the most recent sessions were predictive of change up until that point, indicating that the alliance should be monitored throughout care by the practitioner.

Secondly, and this is a significant result as it pertains directly to rupture–repair outcome correlations. The data in these studies indicate that the alliance scored perfectly 75% of the time, however, those with the best outcomes are not those who necessarily have perfect alliance scores throughout treatment. Our research demonstrated that those who had the best outcomes initially scored lower on the alliance, with the alliance then improving. These findings support the idea that being responsive and attending to ruptures leads to better outcomes, however, the practitioner must have a way to identify such ruptures. For example, in this study, alliance measures were administered at each session. Finally, these data were taken from a naturalistic setting as opposed to a research controlled environment, meaning the results may be more reflective and generalisable to routine practice.

Impact of Alliance Rupture–Repair Training on Outcome

In comparison to the first meta-analysis in this research exploring alliance rupture–repair strategies, the second review examined the correlation between rupture–repair training and client outcomes. While relatively small sample size and study number, the outcomes associated with training tended to be small and not statistically significant. With regard to moderators, several variables in this comparison tend to be related to outcomes. The greater the percentage of patients with personality disorder diagnoses, the smaller the correlation between rupture resolution training and outcome. From a treatment modality perspective, rupture–repair training provided to CBT practitioners tended to be associated with better client outcomes when compared to psychodynamic, as was training provided where treatment duration tended to be shorter. Given the central focus of the alliance in psychodynamic therapy, this finding is not surprising. Other research projects point to attachment style, personality disorders, and motivation for change as being correlated with ruptures (Coutinho, Ribeiro, Fernandes, Sousa, & Safran, 2014; Eames & Roth, 2000). Not addressed in this review, diversity can impact on alliance ruptures, that is, clients who experience microaggressions from their practitioner tend to fair less well in treatment and are at greater risk of drop-out and poorer outcomes (Hook, Davis, Owen, & DeBlaere, 2017).

Top Tips

1. Be attuned to for both withdrawal and conflict ruptures and deal with them immediately in a non-defensive and non-blaming manner.
2. Empathise with the client and accept responsibility for your part in any rupture.
3. If the alliance is not deemed strong enough for explanation of the rupture or if there is another more immediate need, the practitioner can be responsive indirectly by changing the task or exercise to fit these circumstances.
4. The practitioner should consider linking certain interpersonal ruptures to wider issues in the client's life, especially if these ruptures are reflective of the client's way of being in other interpersonal relationships. Be aware that there may be a tendency to use a situation such as this to avoid the immediacy of addressing the difficult ruptures between the practitioner and client by focussing on other relationships.
5. Alliance ruptures can be difficult for practitioners to manage as they can often come with feelings of incompetence, confusion, and guilt. Be aware of these feelings and learn strategies to manage them. In sessions, tolerance of these feelings is especially important if the practitioner is to remain responsive to the client.
6. Practitioners should consider using structured questionnaires to assess the alliance relationship in each session throughout the course of treatment.

Feedback-informed Care

We will recall from the Duncan et al.'s (2010) model that feedback-informed treatment is one of their common factors. The wider literature refers to this way of working in several ways. For example, some call it routine outcome monitoring (ROM), for others, outcome monitoring, another name it goes by is progress feedback. In this chapter, I will be using an all encapsulating term of feedback-informed care. I am using this term to describe the process of collecting information from the client (children, adults, or couples) about their experiences of the process of care (alliance) and their experience of the benefit of treatment (outcome) at each session, and using this information to adapt the treatment approach to the client's needs, wishes, and preferences in real time. That is, being responsive to clients' overall experience by eliciting feedback from them using standardised measures on a session-to-session basis to develop, guide, and evaluate behavioural healthcare interventions and improve outcomes (Brown, Simon, Cameron, & Minami, 2015; Lambert, Whipple, & Kleinstäuber, 2018).

Improving the experience and outcome of care is essential given what we know about the client's experience of therapy. For example, attrition rates are very high overall and average from about 20% (Swift & Greenberg, 2012) to 47% across different outpatient settings (Sparks, Daniels, & Johnson, 2003; Wierzbicki & Pekarik, 1993). Research pertaining to children puts these statistics in a range of 28–85% (Garcia & Weisz, 2002; Kazdin, 1996).

At the same time, approximately 10% of adult clients deteriorate during treatment (Hansen, Lambert, & Forman, 2002); these numbers average about 24% for children and adolescents. However, the research informs us that practitioners tend to be quite poor at identifying those who are not benefiting from care, or indeed those who are deteriorating (Hannan et al., 2005; Hatfield, McCullough, Frantz, & Krieger, 2010; Walfish, McAlister, O'Donnell, & Lambert, 2012) while in our care. Being responsive to these issues through using feedback is one method that can help improve the client's experiences. Critically, using feedback is not about administering measures or questionnaires, it is about creating a culture of feedback with clients in order to become more responsive to their needs. Using feedback can help us learn things about the progress and experience of the client that we would not have learnt otherwise.

Impact of Using Feedback on Outcomes

As noted previously, those not benefiting from care, actively deteriorating or dropping out early make up a large percentage of the average practitioner's caseload. As an evidence based common factor variable, feedback has demonstrated different effectiveness in improving these experiences. The effectiveness of using feedback is dependent on various factors such as the individual practitioner, their training, the level of implementation, their ability to respond to feedback, and the culture of the organisations. As such different studies have demonstrated different effect sizes. In a review of the literature on feedback, Norcross and Lambert (2018) found that the effect sizes differed in the range of d=0.14–0.49. Feedback seems to be most effective for those clients deemed not on track and at risk for deterioration. Meta-analyses conducted in this area tend to have similar findings.

In their meta-analysis of 24 studies with over 8,000 participants using progress feedback, Lambert and Whipple (2018) found that

> two-thirds of the studies found that ROM-assisted psychotherapy was superior to treatment-as-usual offered by the same practitioners .... Feedback practices reduced deterioration rates and nearly doubled clinically significant/reliable change rates in clients who were predicted to have a poor outcome.

While the feedback effect size was small for the overall sample, it was larger for those deemed not on track and at risk for poor outcomes. In the most recent meta-analysis conducted into the use of feedback (de Jong et al., 2021), 58 studies, with a total of 21,699 participants found positive effects for the use of feedback on drop-out rates, number of clients who deteriorated clients, treatment duration, and symptom reduction.

Top Tips

1. Practitioners should solicit feedback from clients using measures of the alliance and outcome of care at each session. Questionnaires should be standardised and reliable.
2. Practitioners should choose the type of outcome measures based on their needs and client population. However, global measure of distress would seem to be most useful for routine practice.
3. Measures should be a means to an end and not an end themselves, practitioners should aim to create a culture of feedback by being responsive.
4. Practitioners should spend the first few minutes of each session discussing scores related to distress, and the last few minutes of each session discussing alliance scores.
5. Practitioners have an ethical obligation to listen to clients' feedback, and change the direction of treatment when indicated to do so.

Conclusion

Cultivating a strong therapeutic alliance is one of the most fundamental jobs of the therapeutic practitioner, and it is strongly predictive of positive outcomes. The bond between the practitioner and client allows the alliance which includes collaborative goal setting to be activated and the tasks of therapy to happen. However, the alliance is a dynamic construct and practitioners must remain vigilant to alliance ruptures which need to be repaired throughout the course of therapy. Soliciting feedback is one way to help repair ruptures, strengthen the alliance, and monitor the outcome of care on a routine basis. These four evidence based relationship factors are pivotal to securing positive outcomes for our clients.

References

Baldwin, S. A., Wampold, B. E., & Imel, Z. E. (2007). Untangling the alliance–outcome correlation: Exploring the relative importance of therapist and patient variability in the alliance. *Journal of Consulting and Clinical Psychology*, *75*(6), 842–852. https://doi.org/10.1037/0022-006X.75.6.842

Bordin, E. S. (1979). The generalizability of the psychoanalytic concept of the working alliance. *Psychotherapy: Theory, Research & Practice*, *16*(3), 252–260. https://doi.org/10.1037/h0085885

Brown, G. S. (J.), Simon, A., Cameron, J., & Minami, T. (2015). A collaborative outcome resource network (ACORN): Tools for increasing the value of psychotherapy. *Psychotherapy*, *52*(4), 412–421. https://doi.org/10.1037/pst0000033

Bordin, E. S. (1979). The generalizability of the psychoanalytic concept of the working alliance. *Psychotherapy: Theory, Research & Practice*, *16*(3), 252–260. https://doi.org/10.1037/h0085885

Coutinho, J., Ribeiro, E., Fernandes, C., Sousa, I., & Safran, J. D. (2014). The development of the therapeutic alliance and the emergence of alliance ruptures. *Anales de Psicología*, *30*, 985–994. http://dx.doi.org/10.6018/analesps.30.3.168911

de Jong, K., Conijn, J. M., Gallagher, R., Reshetnikova, A. S., Heij, M., & Lutz, M. C. (2021). Using progress feedback to improve outcomes and reduce drop-out, treatment duration, and deterioration: A multilevel meta-analysis. *Clinical Psychology Review*, *85*, 102002. https://doi.org/10.1016/j.cpr.2021.102002

Del Re, A. C., Flückiger, C., Horvath, A. O., Symonds, D., & Wampold, B. E. (2012). Therapist effects in the therapeutic alliance–outcome relationship: A restricted-maximum likelihood meta-analysis. *Clinical Psychology Review*, *32*(7), 642–649. https://doi.org/10.1016/j.cpr.2012.07.002

Duncan, B. L., Miller, S. D., Wampold, B. E., & Hubble, M. A. (Eds.). (2010). *American Psychological Association* (2nd ed.). https://doi.org/10.1037/12075-000

Eames, V., & Roth, A. (2000). Patient attachment orientation and the early working alliance: A study of patient and therapist reports of alliance quality and ruptures. *Psychotherapy Research*, *10*(4), 421–434. https://doi.org/10.1093/ptr/10.4.421

Eubanks, C. F., Muran, J. C., & Safran, J. D. (2018). Alliance rupture repair: A meta-analysis. *Psychotherapy*, *55*(4), 508–519. https://doi.org/10.1037/pst0000185

Eubanks, C. F., Sergi, J., & Muran, J. C. (2021). Responsiveness to ruptures and repairs in psychotherapy. In J. C. Watson & H. Wiseman (Eds.), *The responsive psychotherapist: Attuning to clients in the moment* (pp. 83–103). Washington, DC: American Psychological Association. https://doi.org/10.1037/0000240-005

Eubanks-Carter, C., Muran, J. C., & Safran, J. D. (2010). Alliance ruptures and resolution. In J. C. Muran & J. P. Barber (Eds.), *The therapeutic alliance: An evidence-based guide to practice* (pp. 74–94). New York, NY: The Guilford Press.

Flückiger, C., Del Re, A. C., Wampold, B. E., & Horvath, A. O. (2018). The alliance in adult psychotherapy: A meta-analytic synthesis. *Psychotherapy*, *55*(4), 316–340. http://dx.doi.org/10.1037/pst0000172

Flückiger, C., Del Re, A. C., Wlodasch, D., Horvath, A. O., Solomonov, N., & Wampold, B. E. (2020). Assessing the alliance–outcome association adjusted for patient characteristics and treatment processes: A meta-analytic summary of direct comparisons. *Journal of Counseling Psychology*, *67*(6), 706–711. https://doi.org/10.1037/cou0000424

Garcia, J. A., & Weisz, J. R. (2002). When youth mental health care stops: Therapeutic relationship problems and other reasons for ending youth outpatient treatment. *Journal of Consulting and Clinical Psychology*, *70*(2), 439–443. https://doi.org/10.1037/0022-006X.70.2.439

Greenson, R. R. (1965). The working alliance and the transference neuroses. *The Psychoanalytic Quarterly*, *34*, 155–181.

Hook, J. N., Davis, D., Owen, J., & DeBlaere, C. (2017). *Cultural humility: Engaging diverse identities in therapy*. Washington, DC: American Psychological Association. http://dx.doi.org/10.1037/0000037-005

Hannan, C., Lambert, M. J., Harmon, C., Nielsen, S. L., Smart, D. W., Shimokawa, K., & Sutton, S. W. (2005). A lab test and algorithms for identifying clients at risk for treatment failure. *Journal of Clinical Psychology*, *61*(2), 155–163. https://doi.org/10.1002/jclp.20108

Hansen, N. B., Lambert, M. J., & Forman, E. M. (2002). The psychotherapy dose–response effect and its implications for treatment delivery services. *Clinical Psychology: Science and Practice*, *9*(3), 329–343. https://doi.org/10.1093/clipsy.9.3.329

Hatfield, D., McCullough, L., Frantz, S. H., & Krieger, K. (2010). Do we know when our clients get worse? An investigation of therapists' ability to detect negative client change. *Clinical Psychology & Psychotherapy*, *17*(1), 25–32. https://doi.org/10.1002/cpp.656

Kazantzis, N., & Kellis, E. (2012). A special feature on collaboration in psychotherapy. *Journal of Clinical Psychology*, *68*, 133–135. http://dx.doi.org/10.1002/jclp.21837

Kazdin, A. E. (1996). Dropping out of child psychotherapy: Issues for research and implications for practice. *Clinical Child Psychology and Psychiatry*, *1*(1), 133–156. https://doi.org/10.1177/1359104596011012

Lambert, M. J., Whipple, J. L., & Kleinstäuber, M. (2018). Collecting and delivering progress feedback: A meta-analysis of routine outcome monitoring. *Psychotherapy*, *55*(4), 520–537. https://doi.org/10.1037/pst0000167

Mahon, D., Brown, J., & Simon, A. (2021a). The relationship between session-to-session change on a therapeutic alliance measure and outcome of treatment for short term psychotherapy [Web article]. Retrieved from http://www.societyforpsychotherapy.org/the-relationship-between-session-to-session-change-on-a-therapeutic-alliance-measure-and-outcome-of-treatment-for-short-term-psychotherapy

Mahon, D., Brown, J., & Simon, A. (2021b). The relationship between measures of alliance and outcome in psychotherapy lasting more than five sessions [Web article]. Retrieved from http://www.societyforpsychotherapy.org/the-relationship-between-measures-of-alliance-and-outcome-in-psychotherapy-lasting-more-than-five-sessions

Norcross, J. C., & Lambert, M. J. (2018). Psychotherapy relationships that work III. *Psychotherapy*, *55*(4), 303–315. https://doi.org/10.1037/pst0000193

Norcross, J. C., & Lambert, M. J. (2019). Evidence-based psychotherapy relationships: The third task force. In J. C. Norcross & M. J. Lambert (Eds.), *Psychotherapy relationships that work: Evidence-based therapist contributions* (pp. 1–23). Oxford: Oxford University Press. https://doi.org/10.1093/med-psych/9780190843953.003.0001

Safran, J. D., & Muran, J. C. (2000). *Negotiating the therapeutic alliance: A relational treatment guide*. New York, NY: Guilford Press.

Safran, J. D., Muran, J. C., & Eubanks-Carter, C. (2011). Repairing alliance ruptures. In J. C. Norcross (Ed.), Psychotherapy relationships that *work* (2nd ed., pp. 224–238). New York, NY: Oxford University Press. http://dx.doi.org/10.1093/acprof:oso/9780199737208.003.0011

Sparks, W. A., Daniels, J. A., & Johnson, E. (2003). Relationship of referral source, race, and wait time on preintake attrition. *Professional Psychology: Research and Practice*, *34*(5), 514–518. https://doi.org/10.1037/0735-7028.34.5.514

Swift, J. K., & Greenberg, R. P. (2012). Premature discontinuation in adult psychotherapy: A meta-analysis. *Journal of Consulting and Clinical Psychology*, *80*(4), 547–559.

Tryon, G. S., & Winograd, G. (2001). Goal consensus and collaboration. *Psychotherapy*, *38*, 385–389. http://dx.doi.org/10.1037/0033-3204.38.4.385

Tryon, G. S., & Winograd, G. (2011). Goal consensus and collaboration. *Psychotherapy*, *48*, 50–57. http://dx.doi.org/10.1037/a0022061

Tryon, G. S., Birch, S. E., & Verkuilen, J. (2018). Meta-analyses of the relation of goal consensus and collaboration to psychotherapy outcome. *Psychotherapy*, *55*(4), 372–383. https://doi.org/10.1037/pst0000170

Walfish, S., McAlister, B., O'Donnell, P., & Lambert, M. J. (2012). An investigation of self-assessment bias in mental health providers. *Psychological Reports*, *110*(2), 639–644. https://doi.org/10.2466/02.07.17.PR0.110.2.639-644

Wampold, B. E., & Imel, Z. E. (2015). *The great psychotherapy debate* (2nd ed.). London: Routledge/Taylor & Francis Group.

Wierzbicki, M., & Pekarik, G. (1993). A meta-analysis of psychotherapy dropout. *Professional Psychology: Research and Practice*, *24*(2), 190–195. https://doi.org/10.1037/0735-7028.24.2.190

Zetzel, E. R. (1956). Current concepts of transference. *The International Journal of Psychoanalysis*, *37*, 369–376.

Chapter 5

Evidence Based Relationships 2: Treatment Credibility and Outcome Expectancy

Daryl Mahon

Abstract

In the previous chapter, the reader was introduced to four relational common factor variables that impact upon therapy outcomes. In this chapter, I continue the exploration of common factor variables by establishing the research evidence base for another two factors: treatment credibility (TC) and outcome expectancy (OE). The evidence for each individual variable is detailed and Top Tips for each is provided to support both seasoned and beginning practitioners to improve engagement and outcomes. The chapter distinguishes between each of the variables presented, while also acknowledging some overlap and how they complement each other. As with the previous chapter, I have considered these factors together for similar reasons, that is, they are closely aligned and learning about these variables together will help the reader think about how to leverage them in practice.

Keywords: Treatment credibility; outcome expectancy; psychotherapy research; instilling hope; placebo effect; treatment rationale

Chapter Learning Outcomes

(1) Assess the evidence for TC and OE in therapy.
(2) Understand how to leverage these common factors to improve outcomes.

Evidence Based Counselling & Psychotherapy for the 21st Century Practitioner, 53–59

Published under exclusive licence by Emerald Publishing Limited
doi:10.1108/978-1-80455-732-720231005

Introduction

This chapter explores the wider idea of expectations across the therapy experience. Two variables, TC and OE are discussed as essential processes in the therapy experience. TC speaks to the client's belief about how suitable, effective, and logical a treatment may be and is only derived at once the client gains some knowledge about said treatment. Whereas OE reflects the client's prognostic beliefs about the personal efficacy of a planned or current treatment. While TC can only occur in the client once they have been exposed to some knowledge of the treatment, OE can be arrived at before any contact is made between a client and provider.

Although both variables align and there is some overlap, each contributes uniquely to outcomes, and are thus distinct common factors. For example, building TC may well influence OE. The reader will recall from the common factor chapter that building expectancy was discussed across all of the models, although this was done using different terms and concepts.

For example, Wampold's (2015) contextual model illustrates the effect size of expectancy to be about d=0.28, and describes expectancy as occurring in pathway two of the model. Likewise, Grencavage and Norcross (1990) discuss positive expectancy as part of their common factor model, while Lambert (1992) suggested that expectancy contributed approximately 15% of the variance of outcome in his common factor model. Duncan, Hubble, and Miller (2011) discuss expectancy under model delivered/general effects in their common factors. Frank (1961) acknowledges expectancy in the following way: 'A rationale, conceptual scheme, or myth that provides a plausible explanation for the patient's symptoms and prescribes a ritual or procedure for resolving them'. While this latter quote links more so to TC, as opposed to OE, describing both variables under the heading of expectancy provides a good fit for the purpose of this chapter, at least.

Outcome Expectancy

Rosenzweig (1936) was one of the first researchers to acknowledge that expectancy is a common factor. Wampold (2015) describes OE as occurring in pathway two of the contextual model. However, it was Frank (1961) in *Persuasion and Healing* who detailed that clients begin therapy because they are demoralised, and for any therapy to be effective, there must be a mobilisation of belief in the ability to improve. Frank suggests that this positive OE precedes remoralisation, and as such is a trans-theoretical common factor. OE represents the belief about the mental health consequences of participating in psychotherapy. That is, OE is the client's belief in the likely outcome of engaging in a future or current treatment process, it exists on a spectrum of positive to negative. OE can change over the course of treatment based on different factors such as the dynamic of the relationship and influence by therapist factors and treatment experience. While OE may share some commonality with the other factors discussed in this chapter,

Constantino, Coyne, Boswell, Iles, and Vîslă (2018, p. 474) suggest it has been differentiated from:

> Constructs such as patients' treatment expectations, perceptions of treatment or practitioner credibility, treatment motivation, and therapy preferences. Treatment expectations reflect patients' foretelling beliefs about what will transpire during treatment, including how they and their therapist will behave (role expectations), how they will subjectively experience the therapy (process expectations), and how long therapy will last (duration expectation).

OE can manifest in various ways, and while it applies to all people considering therapy, it may present stronger in those who have had prior experiences of therapy (MacNair-Semands, 2002), or those who have strong views on therapy. For example, a client who considers childhood problems to be part of their distress will likely have an OE that will revolve around the need to explore childhood issues in therapy, thus OE is interacting with TC. For example, OE is affected by context, including perhaps most powerfully one's own learning experience. For example, a male client might have had a positive therapy outcome with an older female therapist in the past, which gives him greater faith in the success of a new therapy course if it is recommenced with this same therapist or with a different therapist with salient similarities such as gender, age, or theoretical orientation (Constantino et al., 2018). As we see, OE overlaps significantly with TC, yet both are different concepts. One of the main distinguishing factors of OE is its prognostic outlook.

Impact of OE on Therapy Outcomes

In what was the first meta-analysis of the expectancy–outcomes correlation, Constantino, Glass, Arnkoff, Ametrano, and Smith (2011) using 46 studies which included 8,016 clients demonstrated that OE had a small correlation with outcome of d=0.24. In the most recent meta-analysis, Constantino et al. (2018) included 81 studies with 12,722 clients, and this time the expectancy–outcomes correlation was larger, but still considered a small effect size of d=0.36. Again we can report on some of the mediators and moderators of the OE outcome correlation based on this meta-analysis. Age seemed to somewhat moderate these findings, with a decrease in the correlation as based on age increase. The association also seemed to be stronger where therapy manuals were used or parts of manuals used in comparison to non-manual therapy. Clients with more severe symptoms may be less likely to develop positive OE, while those who report a positive early therapeutic alliance tend to experience more positive OE. Again cultural humility or lack thereof may be one factor that can impact both positively and negatively on the OE, as such practitioners need to consider how OE is related to diversity in their context.

Top Tips

1. Use persuasion when explaining the treatment outcomes rationale. Therapists should draw on how research supports the approach, how the treatment will help the client, and how it meets the criteria for the explanation that the practitioner has provided for the clients presenting issues. Use past success to reinforce these statements.
2. With clients who have low OE or are pessimistic, don't overdo the optimism, rather mirror and show understanding to the clients' plight. Instil hope with statements that do not promise an unrealistic degree of change.
3. Assess the clients' level of OE, checking for visions of unrealistic change.
4. Research suggests that those using or part using manuals have a higher OE outcome correlation. For those who do not use manuals, developing and practicing different rationales and explanations for various presenting problems, and how this will impact outcomes will be beneficial.

Treatment Credibility

A client's belief in the credibility of the treatment process and those providing the treatment is another important common factor. Constantino et al. (2018, p. 486) describe TC as the 'perception of treatment credibility represents their belief about a treatment's personal logicality, suitability, and efficaciousness'. Strong (1968) was among the first to draw on social psychology and articulate that credibility is a determinant of influence, whereby practitioners can build credibility with regard to their professional expertise, trustworthiness, and attractiveness (likeable) to the client. However, almost all the extant literature in this arena examines TC with little to no empirical research of practitioner credibility. Interestingly, a large qualitative study recently established that clients tend to differentiate between TC and practitioner credibility (Finsrud et al., 2022). Devilly and Borkovec (2000) inform us that the client's view of credibility exists on a continuum of positive/negative beliefs regarding the effectiveness and suitability of treatment. However, like OE, TC is a dynamic phenomenon which can change based on interactions with the practitioner and further treatment rationale, assessment and appraisal of therapy, and any improvement in symptoms.

Impact of TC on Outcome

Although the idea of TC has been around for some time, this was largely based on theoretical constructions and single study design. However, we can see the idea of TC within the writings of previously mentioned common factor models.

For example, in Frank's (1961) common factor model, he suggests that there is a need for 'A ritual or procedure that requires the active participation of both patient and therapist and that is believed by both to be the means of restoring the patient's health'. Likewise, Lambert (1992) discusses expectancies and rationale of treatment in his model, while Duncan et al. (2011) speak of the model general effects. Finally, Wampold (2015) suggests that TC occurs in pathway three.

In order to distil the impact of the TC–OE correlation there is only one meta-analysis to date to draw on. Constantino et al. (2018) reviewed the literature based on 24 studies consisting of 1,502 clients, the authors established an effect size of d=0.24. Importantly, the credibility–outcome association seems to be consistent across presenting diagnosis, age, or sex, as well as for treatment orientation, treatment modality type, or whether a treatment manual was or was not used, again indicating its value as a common factor variable. However, some evidence suggests that early symptom improvement can lead to more credibility, while more severe symptoms and distress can lead to lower credibility. There is a paucity of research exploring credibility with more diverse clients, as such, conclusions cannot be drawn.

Top Tips

1. Assess the clients TC at the beginning and throughout therapy having conversations about what clients find compelling about a treatment or task rationale. Likewise assess whether the client sees the practitioner as credible. Client and practitioner characteristics will likely influence whether a client deems a practitioner to be credible to deliver the treatment.
2. Deliver treatment rationale with conviction, this needs to go beyond explaining a treatment protocol and it is thus context specific and needs to be individualised to the presenting issues in the context of the client's story.
3. Be aware of both verbal and non-verbal indications of how the client is receiving the explanation of treatment protocols, be responsive when credibility is low, this can involve offering another treatment modality, adapting modality to better suit the client, or making a referral to another practitioner.
4. Improve client perception of credibility by drawing on what they do find credible, even if this may not be part of the practitioners approach as such. For example, a client might have certain beliefs about the role of medication or faith and the practitioner can encourage this as an adjunct to talk therapy. Or, a client may find only the behavioural aspect of cognitive behavioural therapy (CBT) credible, and thus the practitioner can focus on this.
5. Practitioners should leverage any early change and promote it as evidence that treatment is credible.

Conclusion

TE and OE are important common factors within the therapy space. Unlike the medium to large effect of the variables in the previous chapter, the factors discussed here are of a smaller magnitude. While TC and OE are closely aligned both in research and practice terms, they do represent separate constructs and both influence the outcome of therapy, and as such, practitioners who can leverage these concepts in treatment are more likely to have successful engagement and outcomes. The Top Tips presented alongside each common factor will assist practitioners in their developmental endeavours.

References

Constantino, M. J., Coyne, A. E., Boswell, J. F., Iles, B. R., & Vîslă, A. (2018). A meta-analysis of the association between patients' early perception of treatment credibility and their posttreatment outcomes. *Psychotherapy*, *55*(4), 486–495. https://doi.org/10.1037/pst0000168

Constantino, M. J., Glass, C. R., Arnkoff, D. B., Ametrano, R. M., & Smith, J. Z. (2011). Expectations. In J. C. Norcross (Ed.), *Psychotherapy relationships that work: Evidence-based responsiveness* (2nd ed., pp. 354–376). New York, NY: Oxford University Press. http://dx.doi.org/10.1093/acprof:oso/9780199737208.003.0018

Constantino, M. J., Vîslă, A., Coyne, A. E., & Boswell, J. F. (2018). A meta-analysis of the association between patients' early treatment outcome expectation and their posttreatment outcomes. *Psychotherapy*, *55*(4), 473–485. https://doi.org/10.1037/pst0000169

Devilly, G. J., & Borkovec, T. D. (2000). Psychometric properties of the credibility/expectancy questionnaire. *Journal of Behavior Therapy and Experimental Psychiatry*, *31*, 73–86. http://dx.doi.org/10.1016/S0005-7916(00)00012-4

Duncan, B. L., Hubble, M. A., Miller, S. D. (Eds.). (2011). *The heart & soul of change: Delivering what works in therapy* (2nd ed.). Washington, DC: American Psychological Association.

Finsrud, I., Nissen-Lie, H., Vrabel, K., Høstmælingen, A., Wampold, B., & Ulvenes, P. (2022). It's the therapist and the treatment: The structure of common therapeutic relationship factors. *Psychotherapy Research*, *32*(2), 139–150, doi:10.1080/10503307.2021.1916640

Frank, J. (1961). *Persuasion and healing: A comparative study of psychotherapy*. London: Johns Hopkins University Press.

Grencavage, L. M., & Norcross, J. C. (1990). Where are the commonalities among the therapeutic common factors? *Professional Psychology: Research and Practice*, *21*(5), 372–378. https://doi.org/10.1037/0735-7028.21.5.372

Lambert, M. J. (1992). Psychotherapy outcome research: implications for integrative and eclectic therapists. In J. C. Norcross & M. R. Goldfried (Eds.), *Handbook of psychotherapy integration* (1st ed., pp. 94–129). New York, NY: Basic Books.

MacNair-Semands, R. (2002). Predicting attendance and expectations for group therapy. *Group Dynamics: Theory, Research, and Practice*, *6*, 219–228. http://dx.doi.org/10.1037/1089-2699.6.3.219

Rosenzweig, S. (1936). Some implicit common factors in diverse methods of psychotherapy. *American Journal of Orthopsychiatry*, *6*(3), 412–415. https://doi.org/10.1111/j.1939-0025.1936.tb05248.x

Strong, S. R. (1968). Counseling: An interpersonal influence process. *Journal of Counseling Psychology*, *15*, 215–224. http://dx.doi.org/10.1037/h0020229

Wampold, B. E. (2015). How important are the common factors in psychotherapy? An update. *World Psychiatry: Official Journal of the World Psychiatric Association (WPA)*, *14*(3), 270–277. https://doi.org/10.1002/wps.20238

Chapter 6

Evidence Based Relationships 3: Emotional Expression, Counter-transference, Self-disclosure, and Immediacy

Daryl Mahon

Abstract

In the previous chapter, we explored in a broad sense, the idea of various types of expectancy related to processes involved in the delivery of treatment, and the desire of the client for treatment approaches and other important preferences. In this chapter, I discuss four more variables that we can consider to align to the theme of inner experiences, of the practitioner, with a lesser focus on the client. The relationship between outcomes and emotional expression of the client and practitioner, and outcomes related to the practitioner's counter-transference (CT), self-disclosure (TSD), and use of immediacy (Im) are discussed. As with previous chapter, definitions are provided, the research base is explored, and Top Tips for each variable are outlined for the developing and seasoned practitioner.

Keywords: Emotional expression; counter-transference; self-disclosure; immediacy; psychotherapy processes; psychotherapy variables

Chapter Learning Outcomes

(1) Examine four variables related to the inner experience of the practitioner and client.
(2) Assess a range of strategies for improving responsiveness to clients.

Evidence Based Counselling & Psychotherapy for the 21st Century Practitioner, 61–69

Published under exclusive licence by Emerald Publishing Limited
doi:10.1108/978-1-80455-732-720231006

Introduction

Emotional support is perhaps one of the top reason why individuals seek out the services of a therapeutic practitioner. As such, it is no surprise that emotional expression by the client is an important aspect of therapy, and has a large impact on the outcome of successful care. What may be less known to the average practitioner, is that emotional expression by the practitioner also has an impact on client outcomes. Practitioners sharing their inner experiences is not only considered as it relates to emotional expression, but across several other variables. For example, the practitioner who engages in TSD or Im will often be sharing their inner experience with or about a client in a therapeutic dialogue. In the same vein, much of the information that a practitioner garners about a client comes from their inner reactions to the client in what is described as CT, these inner conflicts are often acted out with the client if the practitioner is not aware of them, or if these issues trigger unresolved conflicts within the practitioner, which can negatively impact therapy outcomes. These four factors are considered below, each involving the sharing of the client and the practitioner of their inner experience.

Emotional Expression

Emotionality is a universal experience and has been at the crux of counselling and psychotherapy theoretical modalities since the emergence of the talking cure. However, it has been only very recent that we have started to understand empirically the relationship between emotional expression and client outcome in therapy (Peluso & Freund, 2018) and emotional work in general (Greenberg, 2016). Emotions are said to have evolved to serve an evolutionary purpose and to assist humans with solving tasks, and to serve a survival purpose by providing information about different circumstance (Ekman, 2007) As such, therapeutic engagement relies on the facilitation and processing of emotional expression in adaptive ways (Greenberg, 2014; Whelton, 2004) which in turn can be used to provide a corrective emotional experience. Practitioners will be familiar with the concept of primary and secondary emotions. What practitioners may largely be unfamiliar with, is that several primary emotions are said to be experienced and expressed the same way regardless of culture, race, or developmental background. Both primary and secondary emotions are influenced by culture, for example, cultural triggers can impact the extent to which a person experiences an emotion and the meaning attached to it can influence the intensity of the emotion (Ekman & Cordaro, 2011), for example, bereavement and grief are experience and expressed in different ways by different cultures.

Emotional processing is a major part of the therapy agenda, and entails organising, making meaning of, and resolving emotional episodes to return to a state of equilibrium (Greenberg, 2016), while emotional regulation entails one's ability to manage and express their emotions adaptively. When discussing the purpose of emotion in therapy, Greenberg (2016, p. 674) argues that emotional processing 'does not involve simply venting emotion, but rather overcoming avoidance of, strongly experiencing, and expressing previously constricted emotions'. As such, both the felt experience and cognitive assessment allows the individual to make meaning of the emotion, in addition to the event or trigger where the original reaction emanated from.

Impact of Emotional Expression on Outcomes

Although there has been no systematic review or meta-analysis of emotional expression–outcome correlation across diverse theoretical orientations, there is research examining various other outcomes related to emotional work, four meta-analyses are of relevance. Orlinsky, Grawe, and Parks (1994) found that therapist focussing on client affect was beneficial in 50% of studies, while both client and practitioner affect were associated with positive outcome in 100% of studies. Diener, Hilsenroth, and Weinberger (2007) found that practitioner facilitation of emotional affect increased client outcomes from 35% to 65% in psychodynamic therapy, while Pascual-Leone and Yeryomenko (2016) found a small effect size for the correlation between client involvement in experiencing new feelings, and outcome of care.

The most recent meta-analysis is the most comprehensive to date, providing two datasets, one for client emotional expression–outcome and another practitioner expression–outcome. Peluso and Freund (2018) conducted two meta-analyses with a total of 66 studies, 13 for practitioners and 43 for clients, which cut across modality and orientation. The 43 client emotional expression meta-analysis had a sample size of 1,715 individuals with a medium to large effect size of d=0.85. For the 16 studies in the second meta-analysis of therapist emotional expression–outcome correlation, the sample consisted of 524 individual's with a medium effect size of d=0.56, indicating that the client's contribution is more important than the practitioners. The study also suggested that there was no moderating effect of client diagnosis, theoretical orientation, outcome measure, or treatment manual, however, none of these proved to be moderators. It is also difficult to draw implications for diversity in this study, other than to note that women outnumbered men two-one, which is a general trend in therapy overall.

Top Tips

1. Emotion matters and practitioners will benefit from finding opportunities to facilitate emotional expression by clients, as opposed to controlling or suppressing them or using techniques to bypass emotions.
2. Suppressing emotions contributes to a negative effect on outcomes. Avoid criticism, dogmatic interpretations, and inflexibility that may promote defensive affect in clients.
3. Practitioners who express affect themselves, contribute to therapeutic outcomes, and facilitate the therapeutic alliance.

4. Practitioners should orientate clients towards emotions, and coach them to learn to manage them. This may mean at times going beyond asking how a client feels, to directing the client to express and then process the cognitive aspects of emotional expression.
5. Practitioners should be aware that emotional processing done in a safe environment can be internalised and used by the client to help regulate emotions. Thus, safety is a key criteria for emotional expression to occur.

TSD and Im

TSD and Im while different constructs, both involve the practitioner reviling something about themselves and their inner world in isolation or in relation to the client. While a controversial topic for classical psychoanalysts who advocate for the blank screen so clients can project their inner world onto the analyst (Greenson, 1967), more recent relational analytical theorists facilitate this by having open dialogue as it relates to the relationship (Levenson, 2010). Of course, humanistic practitioners who focus on genuineness and transparency would view TSD and Im as curative specific factors. Cognitive practitioners will see TSD and Im as being helpful in addressing relationship issues as they arise in therapy. Thus, while some classical analysts may reject aspects of self-disclosure, they have largely trans-theoretical concepts and worthy of research and have clinical utility. Hill and Knox (2002, p. 256) define TSD as:

> Therapist statements that reveal something personal about the therapist … to involve a verbal revelation about the therapist's life outside of therapy. We explicitly excluded from this definition nonverbal self-disclosures … because we sought to focus on verbal statements that therapists share with clients. We also excluded disclosures within or about the therapeutic relationship because we consider these to be Im.

In comparison, Im is about the relationship between the practitioner and client in the here and now, it moves beyond small talk. Or as Kuutmann and Hilsenroth (2012) articulate,

> any discussion within the therapy session about the relationship between therapist and patient that occurs in the here-and-now, as well as any processing of what occurs in the here-and-now patient–therapist interaction.

Of course, Im is often referred to using other terms such as in the here and now work, present centred work, meta-communication, and processing the therapy relationship. Although both concepts involve a disclosure of some sort by the practitioner, they can be differentiated in that TSD are often brief disclosure that do not generate further therapeutic dialogue, whereas Im is more interactive due to its focus on the therapeutic relationship (Pinto-Coelho, Hill, & Kivlighan, 2016).

Impact of TSD and Im on Outcomes

The research into TSD and Im is not as established as some of the factors discussed previously, and the nature of the literature is largely qualitative. Similarly, TSD and Im seem to be used less frequently than other therapy variables. In their review of previous studies, Hill et al. (2018) inform us that previous studies of TSD, reported as being used 0–4% by practitioners, with Im being used between 5 and 38%. Hill and Knox (2002) found that helpful effects of TSD

> Included feeling understood, safer, trusted, comfortable, more open, more present, less protective, special, important, and closer to the therapist ... validated their feelings; helped them feel better outside of therapy ...; and changed how clients saw the therapist by fostering trust in the therapist, equalizing the relationship, enabling clients to see the therapist as a real person, and making it easier to talk to the therapist.

TSD and Im may not always be experienced as favourable by clients. In a review of 14 studies, Ackerman and Hilsenroth (2001) found that when TSD revealed too much of the practitioner's own conflicts, it could weaken the alliance and boundaries. In a qualitative meta-analysis of 21 studies, Hill et al. (2018) explicated that TSD was a predictor of improved client mental health and therapy relationship, and benefits for insight, while Im was a predictor of clients opening up and disclosing and enhancing the therapeutic relationship. The findings are largely positive from this review, however, approximately 30% of cases found a negative effect meaning practitioners need to be cautious in how they go about utilising TSD and Im. There is still a way to go with regard to research in TSD and Im, and while there is not enough research to draw conclusion on diversity factors, two possible issues are important to note. That is, for some cultures, Im may feel rude or indeed threatening, while for some minoritised clients, practitioner TSD can be helpful to build trust and safety.

Top Tips

1. Practitioners from all orientations should consider using TSD and Im. However, this should be done sparingly and thoughtfully.

2. When considering using TSD practitioners should use it in the context of the client's current difficulties to facilitate client exploration. Judicial and well timed TSD can help clients understand the universality of human suffering and distress.
3. Im is best used in the context of the therapy relationship to process emotions and feelings regarding the alliance. However, this may also magnify ruptures, so practitioners need to be aware of this, and be able to manage these feeling and processes.
4. Practitioners should be attentive when using both TSD and Im. The research indicates that not all clients respond favourably to these processes. Be aware of client responses, non-verbal behaviour, and enquire as to the experience. This is best done within a well-developed and robust therapeutic alliance.

Managing CT

As with many psychotherapy processes and concepts, CT can be traced back to the dawn of psychotherapy, and the work of Sigmond Freud. For the classical analyst, CT was something to be controlled, not discussed as practitioners were expected to remain as the blank slate for the client to project onto. However, CT is a trans-theoretical construct that shows up in all therapeutic relationships. There are perhaps three main conceptions of CT, classical, totalistic, and complementary, found in the literature (Epstein & Feiner, 1988). Freud (1910/1957) posited that classical CT is an unconscious process on the part of the practitioner that is rooted in unresolved childhood conflicts which are triggered by the client's transference. These manifestations are seen by classicals as interrupting the psychotherapy process. In comparison, the totalistic definition of CT suggests that all reactions that a practitioner have towards a client are transference which can orientate the practitioner to important information that can be used for therapeutic understanding through reflection and examination (Heimann, 1960). The final type of CT emanates from interpersonal and object relations psychoanalytical thought. Complementary CT is said to occur in relation to the client's way of relating. For example, the client who continues to feel powerlessness in their life may tend to generate feelings of powerlessness in the practitioner with regard to assisting the client.

Hayes, Gelso, Goldberg, and Kivlighan (2018) suggest that CT needs to have some conceptual definition to study it, and as such find an integrative definition that is narrower than the totalistic one. Thus, they operationalise CT as 'as internal and external reactions in which unresolved conflicts of the therapist, usually but not always unconscious, are implicated' (p. 497). Thus, this definition has clinical utility not such for transference reactions, but also for reactions to other client factors such as personality, how the client presents, their personal problems, and their worldview. As such it is something that all practitioners experience, regardless of modality.

Impact of CT on Outcomes

Thus far, studies in the extant literature have focussed on the CT phenomena and associated outcomes from several differentiated perspectives. The following three CT outcome correlations have been researched enough to contribute to meta-analysis:

(1) The association between CT reactions and psychotherapy outcome.
(2) The relationship between CT reactions and CT management.
(3) The association between CT management and psychotherapy outcome.

Findings from recent studies were mixed overall, which is not surprising considering the direction of the research and the different correlations explored (Hayes & Cruz, 2006; Hayes, Gelso, & Hummel, 2011). The most recent review conducted by Hayes et al. (2018) included three different meta-analyses that examined the relationship with CT and outcome of therapy, CT management and the relationship with CT reactions, and CT management and better therapy outcomes.

In the first meta-analysis, which included 14 studies and 973 participants with a small to moderate effect size of d=0.33, is consistent with a previous meta-analysis with less studies. This finding indicates that more frequent CT reactions are associated with worse therapy outcomes. The second meta-analysis explored the relationship between CT management and CT reactions, which included 13 studies with 1,394 participants and found a moderate relationship with effect size of d=0.55, demonstrating that more effective CT management is associated with fewer reactions. Finally, 9 studies with 392 participants indicate that CT management and its relationship with therapy outcomes has a large effect size of d=0.84. Less is known about the cultural implications of CT, however, research across cultural humility and orientation would indicate that differences in outcomes when working with diverse identities could be a function of CT. While in general terms, there have been no client characteristics identified that are predictive of CT in the practitioner, demonstrating the idiosyncratic nature of CT. As such, Hayes et al. (2018, p. 504) suggest that 'it is incumbent upon therapists to understand themselves, their own inner workings, and to know what types of clients will likely provoke their CT reactions'.

Top Tips

1. Practitioners should take seriously the impact CT can have on therapy, as such practitioners will benefit from building self-awareness and insight into their inner worlds, practicing self-appraisal and self-observation.
2. Practitioners of all orientations will find self-integration especially helpful to mitigate CT, thus personal therapy may be helpful. While CT

happens with all practitioners, chronic reoccurring CT may be a good indicator of internal/unconscious conflicts that need to be resolved.

3. Practitioners can develop their emotional capacity and regulation skills by engaging in meditation. Other self-care strategies such as, mindfulness, diet, sleep, and exercise will also be beneficial.
4. Supervision is another area where practitioners can engage in to support the management and identification of CT.
5. When CT reactions have been acted upon with the client, acknowledging this is needed, and rupture–repair strategies need to be applied. Practitioners do not need to go into details of the CT conflicts but acknowledging these with the client is helpful.

Conclusion

The processing of client emotions is one of the most fundamental tasks of therapy and clients who express emotions in therapy tend to have more favourable outcomes. At the same time, practitioners who express their emotions to clients also impact positively on the outcome of therapy. It is not just emotions that practitioners can express to help the therapy process along, other aspects of the practitioner's inner world can be used as an impetus for change. For example, using TSD, and by using Im in the relationship, as a here and now process both have demonstrated to be powerful evidence based relationship variables. However, not all the practitioner's inner experiences are positive, and some need to be managed, such as CT. Despite this, if dealt with correctly, CT management is associated with better therapy outcomes, and as such, strategies to achieve this are recommended.

References

Ackerman, S. J., & Hilsenroth, M. J. (2001). A review of therapist characteristics and techniques negatively impacting the therapeutic alliance. *Psychotherapy*, *38*, 171–185. http://dx.doi.org/10.1037/0033-3204.38.2.171

Diener, M. J., Hilsenroth, M. J., & Weinberger, J. (2007). Therapist affect focus and patient outcomes in psychodynamic psychotherapy: A meta analysis. *The American Journal of Psychiatry*, *164*, 936–941. http://dx.doi.org/10.1176/ajp.2007.164.6.936

Ekman, P. (2007). *Emotions revealed. Second edition: Recognizing faces and feelings to improve communication and emotional life*. New York, NY: Henry Holt and Company, LLC.

Ekman, P., & Cordaro, D. (2011). What is meant by calling emotions basic? *Emotion Review*, *3*, 364–370. http://dx.doi.org/10.1177/1754073911410740

Epstein, L., & Feiner, A. H. (1988). Countertransference: The therapist's contribution to treatment. In B. Wolstein (Ed.), *Essential papers on countertransference* (pp. 282–303). New York, NY: New York University Press.

Freud, S. (1910/1957). Future prospects of psychoanalytic therapy. In J. Strachey (Ed.), *The standard edition of the complete works of Sigmund Freud* (Vol. 11, pp. 139–151). London: Hogarth Press.

Greenberg, L. S. (2014). The therapeutic relationship in emotion-focused therapy. *Psychotherapy*, *51*, 350–357. http://dx.doi.org/10.1037/a0037336

Hayes, J. A., & Cruz, J. M. (2006). On leading a horse to water: Therapist insight, countertransference, and client insight. In L. G. Castonguay & C. E. Hill (Eds.), *Insight in psychotherapy* (pp. 279–292). Washington, DC: American Psychological Association.

Hayes, J. A., Gelso, C. J., & Hummel, A. M. (2011). Managing countertransference. In J. C. Norcross (Ed.), *Psychotherapy relationships that work* (2nd ed., pp. 239–258). New York, NY: Oxford University Press. http://dx.doi.org/10.1093/acprof:oso/9780199737208.003.0012

Hayes, J. A., Gelso, C. J., Goldberg, S., & Kivlighan, D. M. (2018). Countertransference management and effective psychotherapy: Meta-analytic findings. *Psychotherapy*, *55*(4), 496–507. https://doi.org/10.1037/pst0000189

Heimann, P. (1960). Counter-transference. *The British Journal of Medical Psychology*, *33*, 9–15. http://dx.doi.org/10.1111/j.2044-8341.1960.tb01219.x

Hill, C. E., & Knox, S. (2002). Self-disclosure. *Psychotherapy*, *38*, 412–416.

Hill, C. E., Knox, S., & Pinto-Coelho, K. G. (2018). Therapist self-disclosure and immediacy: A qualitative meta-analysis. *Psychotherapy*, *55*(4), 445–460. https://doi.org/10.1037/pst0000182

Kuutmann, K., & Hilsenroth, M. J. (2012). Exploring in-session focus on the patient-therapist relationship: Patient characteristics, process and outcome. *Clinical Psychology and Psychotherapy*, *19*, 187–202. http://dx.doi.org/10.1002/cpp.743

Levenson, H. (2010). *Brief dynamic therapy*. Washington, DC: American Psychological Association.

Leslie S. G. (2017). Emotion-focused therapy of depression. *Person-Centered & Experiential Psychotherapies*, *16*(2), 106–117, doi: 10.1080/14779757.2017.1330702

Orlinsky, D. E., Grawe, K., & Parks, B. K. (1994). Process and outcome in psychotherapy. In A. E. Bergin & S. L. Garfield (Eds.), *Handbook of psychotherapy and behavior change* (4th ed., pp. 270–376). New York, NY: Wiley.

Pascual-Leone, A., & Yeryomenko, N. (2016). The client "experiencing" scale as a predictor of treatment outcomes: A meta-analysis on psychotherapy process. *Psychotherapy Research*, *27*, 653–665. http://dx.doi.org/10.1080/10503307.2016.1152409

Peluso, P. R., & Freund, R. R. (2018). Therapist and client emotional expression and psychotherapy outcomes: A meta-analysis. *Psychotherapy*, *55*(4), 461–472. https://doi.org/10.1037/pst0000165

Pinto-Coelho, K., Hill, C. E., & Kivlighan, D., Jr. (2016). Therapist self-disclosures in psychodynamic psychotherapy: A mixed methods investigation. *Counselling Psychology Quarterly*, *29*, 29–52. http://dx.doi.org/10.1080/09515070.2015.1072496

Whelton, W. J. (2004). Emotional processes in psychotherapy: Evidence across therapeutic modalities. *Clinical Psychology and Psychotherapy*, *11*, 58–71. http://dx.doi.org/10.1002/cpp.392

Chapter 7

Evidence Based Relationships 4: Empathy, Congruence, Unconditional Positive Regard, and Real Relationship

Daryl Mahon

Abstract

The last chapter examined evidence based relationships from the perspective of emotional expression and the inner experience of the practitioner in relation to the client. In this chapter, I am introducing the first of a number of variables situated in evidence based relationships. Empathy, congruence, unconditional positive regard, and the real relationship will be discussed. I have chosen to categorise these four variables together due to their significant overlap and interaction with each other in terms of practice and research. This chapter does not attempt to provide an exhaustive description of each factor. Rather, I provide a very brief overview of the variable, provide an analysis of the research behind each, and highlight Top Tips that can guide the practitioner in their development.

Keywords: Empathy; congruence; unconditional positive regard; real relationships; psychotherapy variables; evidence based relationships

Chapter Learning Outcomes

(1) Assess the evidence for several relationship variables.
(2) Identify areas for further development based on four common factors.

Evidence Based Counselling & Psychotherapy for the 21st Century Practitioner, 71–83

Published under exclusive licence by Emerald Publishing Limited
doi:10.1108/978-1-80455-732-720231007

Introduction

This is the first chapter addressing various components of psychotherapy and assessing their impact on and contribution to therapy outcomes. The variables discussed in this and subsequent chapters can be considered to sit within the common factors of therapy. While some will be recognisable from the Wampold contextual model discussed previously, not all of them are found in that model. I include other variables identified by researchers Norcross and Lambert (2018) as being effective evidence based relationship factors.

Both the beginning and seasoned therapist alike will be familiar with the four variables in this chapter as three of them are the main core conditions in Carl Rogers's person-centred therapy (PCT). However, Carl Rogers's PCT is a comprehensive theory of personality based on humanistic thinking, and what we are discussing in this chapter is different variables that cut across various theories. That is, this is not a chapter about PCT, it is about the variables as stand-alone evidence based practices. As those of you practicing will realise, the evidence based relationship factors are hugely impactful. However, unlike theory and techniques, they are not competencies that can be taught in a standardised way. Rather, how a practitioner responds with empathy or unconditional, for example, will depend on the client and their story, the practitioners worldview, awareness, development, experiential avoidance, and counter-transference. Thus, the response one practitioner gives to a client may be quite different than the response another practitioner may give to the same client. However, there is guidance that we can take from the research literature with regard to general principles and best practices.

Empathy

As articulated previously, this chapter is not about PCT, or about any model of therapy, it is about different individual variables that impact on client outcomes across modalities. That being said, it would be amiss to not mention Carl Rogers and his work during the 1940s–1950s, especially as it relates to empathy. While empathy is a relational component of all successful therapy, Rogers and his colleagues were perhaps the first to codify and position it as an essential helping skill. After a relatively long period without much empirical investigation, empathy was taken back by academics across various fields such as neuroscience (Decety & Ickes, 2009) and medicine where it has shown to make medical procedures more effective (Pedersen, 2009). Most practitioners will have taken their understanding and conception of empathy from Carl Rogers, and I find his following definition of accurate empathy to be useful, insightful, and descriptive. Rogers (1959, p. 210) describes accurate empathy as:

> The state of empathy, or being empathic, is to perceive the internal frame of reference of another with accuracy and with the emotional components and meanings which pertain thereto as if one were the person, but without ever losing the 'as if' condition. Thus it means to sense the hurt or the pleasure of another as he

> senses it and to perceive the causes thereof as he perceives them, but without ever losing the recognition that it is as if I were hurt or pleased and so forth. If this 'as if' quality is lost, then the state is one of identification.

However, there are lots of other definitions and conceptions of empathy, and while not the purpose of this chapter to provide an operationalisation and definition, it would be wrong to not mention the wide range of researchers who have contributed to our understanding of this construct. For example, Barrett-Lennard (1981), Egan (1982), and Truax and Carkhuff (1967) have all contributed to and defined empathy. In a review of definitions in their meta-analysis, Elliott, Bohart, Watson, and Murphy (2018) provide the following definitions and operationalisations:

1. Empathy is interpersonal and unidirectional, provided by one person to another person.
2. Empathy is conceptualized primarily as an ability or capacity, and occasionally as an action.
3. Empathy involves a range of related mental abilities/actions, such as
   3.1. Primarily: Understanding the other person's feelings, perspectives, experiences, or motivations
   3.2. Awareness of, appreciation of, or sensitivity to, the other person
   3.3. Gained through: Active entry into the other's experience, described variously in terms of vicariousness, imagination, sharing, or identification.

Levels of Empathy

Empathy has also been defined and operationalised in terms of differential levels. The Traux and Carkhuff's (1967) empathy rating scale proposes and measures empathy on a scale from 1 to 5. This is an important framework for the novice and seasoned practitioner to be aware of as it can act as a structured guide in helping to advance empathy skills. Table 5 provides an overview and description of levels 1–5. Crucially, the levels of empathy go beyond the idea that this construct is generally only about reflecting on feelings, as it is much more than this. Elliott et al. (2018, p. 400) provide the following analysis of this argument:

> Interestingly, the two therapeutic approaches that have most focused-on empathy – person-centred therapy and psychoanalytic therapy – have emphasized its cognitive or perspective-taking aspects ... focusing mainly on understanding the client's frame of reference or way of experiencing the world. By some accounts, 70% or more of Carl Rogers's responses were to felt meaning rather than to feeling, despite the fact that his mode of responding is typically described as reflection of feeling.

Table 5. Five Levels of Empathy.

Empathy level	Description
Level 1: Low level of responding	Practitioner communicates no awareness or understanding, advise provided, and subject changed responses are irrelevant
Level 2: Moderate low level of responding	Practitioners show some effort, surface level understanding, wrong interpretation of emptions, and feelings omitted from responses
Level 3: Interchangeable level of responding	Practitioners demonstrate both verbal and non-verbal responses that accurately capture the surface feelings and client's story
Level 4: Moderately high responding	Are aimed at developing client self-awareness. Practitioners identify implicit underlying feelings, the practitioner identifies nuances and aspects of the emotions, meanings, and behaviours, including unexplored feelings
Level 5: High level of responding	Practitioners reflect emotional nuances, they mirror voice and intensity of expression to the client moment by moment. Both surface and implicit feelings and meaning are captured. Feelings and meanings are often connected to previous life experiences, examining themes and life patterns. Implicit goals which can provide direction for personal growth are identified in the client's message

Impact of Empathy on Outcomes

As discussed at the outset of this chapter, empathy as an evidence based relationship variable has a big impact on the outcome of psychotherapy. Two previous meta-analyses demonstrated that empathy has a moderate impact on client outcomes (Bohart, Elliott, Greenberg, & Watson, 2002; Elliott, Bohart, Watson, & Greenberg, 2011). In the most recent meta-analysis built on the previous mentioned studies and reviewing 82 articles involving 6,138 clients, Elliott et al. (2018) found that empathy is a moderately strong predictor of client outcomes, with a Cohens *d* of 0.58. Some interesting findings from this review suggest that this effectiveness was consistent across theoretical modalities, and client presenting problems, which of course supports the common factor proposition. Overall empathy is said to account for approximately 9% of the variance in outcomes. However, there was high heterogeneity in the overall effects, and this may speak to the ability of individual practitioners in expressing empathy. That is, some practitioners are clearly more effective in responding to clients in empathic ways. Practitioners new to the field and those who are already well established will likely have room to improve in this important common factor. The following Top Tips provide practitioners seeking to improve their empathic responses with some guidance and direction.

Top Tips

1. Practitioners must be attuned to the impact and meaning of clients' stories, not necessarily the words or content, although capturing the content is important.
2. Practitioners must hold their assumptions lightly and be willing to change and adapt their empathic response based on the clients' reactions.
3. Practitioners aiming for high levels of empathic responses must attend to implicit meaning and feelings on the edge of the clients awareness
4. Practitioners who co-create high levels of empathy understand their clients' goals, wishes, and needs, and can respond to nuances and in the context of the clients' previous life experiences.
5. Empathy is closely related to other relational evidence based factors such as unconditionality and congruence and should be provided in the context of these authentic relational variables.

Unconditional Positive Regard

Unconditional positive regard is another powerful common factor variable that has been demonstrated to be predictive of successful therapy. Much like empathy however, there are often different definitions used to describe it. Practitioners may be familiar with or use some of the following words when describing positive regard. For example, affirmation, respect, non-possessive warmth, support, validation, and prizing the client. Again, unconditionality is one of the core conditions of Carl Rogers and so it may be instructive to return to Rogers for a description.

> To the extent that the therapist finds himself experiencing a warm acceptance of each aspect of the client's experience as being a part of that client, he is experiencing unconditional positive regard .... It means there are no conditions of acceptance .... It means a 'prizing' of the person ... it means a caring for the client as a separate person. (Rogers, 1957, p. 101)

While this is but one of Rogers descriptions, it seems to cover the concept nicely, while at the same time helping us to understand how positive regard is a common factor that crosses theoretical orientations. Breger (2009) provides a useful story about Freud and psychoanalysis, and how positive regard seems to be a heart of successful therapy.

> When Freud followed these [psychoanalytic] rules his patients did not make progress. His well-known published cases are failures … in contrast are patients like Kardiner and others – cases he never wrote or publicly spoke about – all of whom found their analyses very helpful. With these patients, what was curative was not neutrality, abstinence, or interpretations of resistance, but a more open and supportive relationship, interpretations that fit their unique experiences, empathy, praise, and the feelings that they were liked by their analyst. (p. 105)

These deep human needs, wishes, and desires that are most personal, also tend to be universal and I feel the need to invoke, once again, one of the great relational psychotherapists of our time to demonstrate what unconditional positive regard might look like when being expressed to a client. In the below scenario, Yalom is responding to a client who considers Yalom to have negative feelings towards them …

> You're reading me entirely wrong. I don't have any of those feelings. I've been pleased with our work. You've shown a lot of courage, you work hard, you've never missed a session, you've never been late, you've taken chances by sharing so many intimate things with me. In every way here, you do your job. But I do notice that whenever you venture a guess about how I feel about you, it often does not jibe with my inner experience, and the error is always in the same direction: You read me as caring for you much less than I do. (Yalom, 2002, p. 24)

Impact of Unconditional Positive Regard on Outcomes

Like other psychotherapy relationship factors, unconditionality has a small to moderate impact on outcomes. Orlinsky, Grawe, and Parks (1994) studied positive regard naming it therapist affirmation and found it to be a significant factor, but with mixed effect sizes. Farber and Doolin (2011) found that when the client rated the therapist's positive regard and outcome, a positive trend occurred, while moderate effect sizes were found on treatment outcome and larger effect sizes were found for treatment retention. In a meta-analysis, Farber and Doolin (2011) once again demonstrated that positive regard has a moderate effect on psychotherapy outcomes and that it accounts for about 9% of the variance of outcomes in psychotherapy.

In their most recent meta-analysis with 68 studies which included 3,528 individuals, Farber and Doolin (2018) updated and extended findings from previous reviews. This review included studies across modes, models, and settings, in addition to different groups of people such as adults, children, family, and group therapy. They surmise that this may be one reason for the smaller effect size than noted in previous reviews. Examining possible moderators of positive regard, the authors suggest that:

> positive regard tends to have a more powerful association with psychotherapy outcome in individual therapy, in an outpatient setting, when therapy is performed by trainees, with clients presenting with mood or anxiety disorders (as opposed to severe mental illness), and when outcome is assessed via measures of global or overall symptomatology, as opposed to specific indices of depression or anxiety. (p. 417)

The authors suggest that positive regard is more effective with anxieties and depression as opposed to more serious psychopathology, supporting Rogers's (1957) initial view of positive regard when working with Schizophrenia as not being effective.

Top Tips

1. Provide positive regard, for some it may be sufficient, while it also interacts and overlaps with other evidence based factors such as empathy and congruence. It is unlikely that it operates in isolation.
2. Keep in mind that affirming clients may serve a function in helping the client engage in therapy, help self-disclosure, provide a foundation for the client to engage in relationships, and facilitates resilience and growth.
3. Don't just feel positive regard, express it. This does not and probably should not be expressed as running compliments, as this may negatively impact clients. Rather, expressing a deep caring consistently for the client is how positive regard should be expressed.
4. Positive regard can be conveyed in various ways. Caring words, creating positive narratives, active listening, flexibility in scheduling, speaking in a gentle tone of voice, establishing responsive eye contact, and maintaining positive body language.
5. Practitioners will vary in their ability to convey positive regard, as will clients' needs to receive it. Practitioners need to be aware of this and monitor both cases. Many ruptures to the alliance can happen through practitioners not monitoring this important aspect of therapy.
6. Use supervision to reflect on how you convey positive regard, potential blocks, and the likely outcomes or lack of outcomes.

Congruence

The next variable we examine is congruence or genuineness as it is often referred to as. Once again, this variable is probably most associated with the person-centred work of Carl Rogers who first described and codified this relational common factor. While congruence is often recognised as belonging to the person centre tradition, it is also of value to other modalities although not always articulated as such, and thus, it is a common factor. Kolden, Wang, Austin, Chang, and Klein (2018) describe congruence in the following way:

> Congruence is an aspect of the therapy relationship with two facets, one intrapersonal and one interpersonal. Mindful genuineness, personal awareness, and authenticity characterize the intrapersonal element. The capacity to respectfully and transparently give voice to ones' experience to another person characterizes the interpersonal component. (p. 424)

While Rogers (1957) proposed that for congruence to be effective as a therapeutic process, the client must be in a state of incongruence. While the practitioner must be congruent based on two fundamental elements. Namely, the practitioner must be freely and deeply him or herself, while having the skill to convey this state to the client. Barrett-Lennard (1998) extended this understanding by emphasising the client's perception of congruence as being the essential factor in the outcome of therapy. As with empathy, we cannot really discuss congruence without mentioning the other relationship variables that overlap and interact with congruence. Empathy, positive regard, and the real relationship are closely related. Indeed, Kolden et al. (2018, p. 424) inform us that 'Congruence plays a central role in this framework, in that it is a prerequisite for the transmission of empathy and positive regard'.

Impact of Congruence on Outcomes

The congruence outcome correlation has been researched in meta-analyses going back as far as 1973 and thus far there has been 16 conducted with mixed results. For the purpose of this chapter, the results from the last three meta-analyses seem most pertinent, considering the advances in methodology since 1973. In a meta-analysis examining 16 studies with 863 clients, Kolden, Klein, Wang, and Austin (2011) found the congruence–outcome correlation to be small to moderate with d=0.48, which means congruence contributes to about 6% of the variance of outcomes in psychotherapy. In their most recent meta-analysis, Kolden et al. (2018) with 21 studies and 1,192 clients, the findings were just slightly smaller than the previous meta-analysis with a finding of d=0.46, corresponding to a contribution of 5.3% to the variance in psychotherapy outcome.

When examining possible moderators of the congruence outcome correlation, the Kolden et al.'s (2018) study found some interesting moderators, many were also identified in previous meta-analyses. The age of the practitioner, clinical experience, and licenced practitioners as opposed to trainees all showed positive correlations on the congruence outcome of therapy. Younger age and college counselling settings also produced more positive correlations compared to older adults, and those using clinical psychiatry services, while there was no findings for gender or educational attainment. There was no difference between modality, although previous meta-analysis showed psychodynamic to have a stronger correlation with congruence outcome when exploring it from a theoretical perspective.

Top Tips

1. Practitioners will be best served by 'owning their feelings'. This act of intentional genuineness can be operationalist with regard to the client by voicing their thoughts and feelings about an interaction they had with the client, or how they're are experiencing the client. Congruence is not a free for all say what you like concept, it needs to be in relation to the client.
2. Congruence can act as the vehicle in which empathy and positive regard is framed, it does not act in isolation.
3. Therapists can model congruence in sessions. A variety of skills might be brought to bear to accomplish this. Congruent responding includes moderated self-disclosure of personal information and life experiences. It could also entail articulation of thoughts and feelings, opinions, pointed questions, and feedback regarding patient behaviour. Genuine responses are honest. Congruent responses are not disrespectful, overly intellectualised .... Genuine therapist responses are cast in the language of personal pronouns (Kolden et al., 2018).
4. Clients may need different types and level of congruence and practitioners should monitor and reflect on how they achieve this.

The Real Relationship

While the previous three variables discussed thus far are mostly associated with Carl Rogers, the real relationship can be traced back to the work of Sigmond Freud (1937, p. 222) who postulated that

> not every relation between an analyst and his subject during and after analysis was to be regarded as transference; there were also friendly relations which were based on reality and proved to be viable.

Freud was not the only analyst to speak of the real relationship, indeed his daughter Anna Freud also spoke of its importance, as did Greenson (1967) who built on this concept by adding genuineness and realism to it. As we can see, the real relationship is closely aligned to the other constructs discussed in this chapter. In fact, Gelso, Kivlighan, and Markin (2018, p. 434) conceptualised it in the following:

> The real relationship is the personal relationship between patient and therapist marked by the extent to which each is genuine with the other and perceives/experiences the other in ways that are realistic. The strength of the real relationship is determined by both the extent to which it exists and the degree to which it is positive or favourable.

Again, we can see that the real relationship is a trans-theoretical common factor, and empirical research has demonstrated that it is not related to one's theoretical orientation (Gelso, 2011). Research suggests that three other psychotherapy constructs are closely related to the real relationship, the therapeutic alliance, client transference, and client and therapist attachment. It is beyond this chapter to delve into these other key relationship factors, although the alliance and transference are explored more in subsequent chapters.

Impact of the Real Relationship on Outcomes

To date there has only been one meta-analysis conducted that has examined the real relationship–outcome correction. Gelso et al. (2018) meta-analysed 16 studies with 1,502 individual clients and indicated a moderate to large effect size for the real relationship–outcome correlation. The outcome association was independent of the type of outcome assessed, for example, treatment outcomes, session outcomes, and treatment progress. When exploring possible moderators of the real relationship on outcomes, findings suggest that the therapists' contribution is more important than the clients, and that this contribution is related to decreases in symptoms across treatment. The clients' contribution to the real relationship is also important, with clients who can see and experience the practitioner as s/he really is and those who can stand back and view themselves objectively better able to engage in the real relationship. Clients who tend to avoid their inner feelings are also less likely to engage in the real relationship, while those who tend to securely attach have been found to be more likely to engage the real relationship. One point to note, emerging research suggests practitioners who display a multicultural orientation working within diversity are more likely to develop stronger real relationship (Owen, Tao, Leach, & Rodolfa, 2011). Ravind Jeawon and I discuss this concept in a later chapter on multicultural practices. While the research suggests that the real relationship changes across the course of treatment, with bonds developing more strongly, there is also practices and attitudes that the practitioner can adopt to help facilitate this process in a more timely manner, or indeed at times when the practitioner is having difficulty cultivating the real relationship.

Top Tips

1. Accurate empathy is one way to help establish the real relationship. Accurate empathy can help facilitate the realism aspect for the practitioner, and help model empathy for the client, who in turn may then start to experience the practitioner in a more realistic light.
2. Tending to counter-transference by the practitioner managing their anxieties, boundaries, and self-awareness and being genuine with the client can all help cultivate the real relationship.
3. Practitioner self-disclosure is related to the real relationship through the act of being genuine. While disclosures if being made should be for the benefit of the client and relate to the therapy relationship, they can help the client experience the practitioner as more genuine.
4. Informing the client that one is not willing to self-disclose is paradoxically a form of self-disclosure and thus will also help the client to experience the practitioner as being genuine. Practitioners should explain in straight forward terms why they are not disclosing.
5. Being consistent with clients is integral. Practitioners demonstrate this through verbal and non-verbal behaviour. Consistency encourages trust, and lets the client know that the practitioner can be trusted and is reliable.

Conclusion

Developing evidence based relationship skills is not without its complications. Unlike theories and techniques in psychotherapy, relational factors can't be standardised and are thus more difficult to develop. The four common factors discussed in this chapter each play an important role in effective psychotherapy outcomes, although we must acknowledge the correlation not causality dimension. There is a great deal of overlap in the four factors, and the research suggests that they don't exist in a vacuum. The Top Tips presented for each common factor will help the novice and seasoned practitioner to hone their skills through a concerted effort and by practicing at the edge of their growth level.

References

Barrett-Lennard, G. T. (1981). The empathy cycle: Refinement of a nuclear concept. *Journal of Counseling Psychology*, *28*, 91–100. http://dx.doi.org/10.1037/0022-0167.28.2.91

Barrett-Lennard, G. T. (1998). *Carl Rogers' helping system: Journey and substance*. Beverly Hills, CA: Sage.

Breger, L. (2009). *A dream of undying fame: How Freud betrayed his mentor and invented psychoanalysis*. New York, NY: Basic Books.

Bohart, A. C., Elliott, R., Greenberg, L. S., & Watson, J. C. (2002). Empathy. In J. Norcross (Ed.), *Psychotherapy relationships that work* (pp. 89–108). New York, NY: Oxford University Press.

Decety, J., & Ickes, W. (Eds.). (2009). *The social neuroscience of empathy*. Cambridge, MA: MIT Press. http://dx.doi.org/10.7551/mitpress/9780262012973.001.0001

Egan, G. (1982). *The skilled helper* (2nd ed.). Monterey, CA: Brooks/Cole.

Elliott, R., Bohart, A. C., Watson, J. C., & Greenberg, L. S. (2011). Empathy. In J. Norcross (Ed.), *Psychotherapy relationships that work* (2nd ed., pp. 132–152). New York, NY: Oxford University Press. http://dx.doi.org/10.1093/acprof:oso/9780199737208.003.0006

Elliott, R., Bohart, A. C., Watson, J. C., & Murphy, D. (2018). Therapist empathy and client outcome: An updated meta-analysis. *Psychotherapy*, *55*(4), 399–410. https://doi.org/10.1037/pst0000175

Farber, B. A., & Doolin, E. M. (2011). Positive regard. *Psychotherapy*, *48*(1), 58–64. https://doi.org/10.1037/a0022141

Freud, S. (1937). Analysis terminable and interminable. In J. Stratchy (Ed.), *Standard edition of the complete works of Sigmund Freud* (pp. 209–253). London: Hogarth Press.

Gelso, C. J. (2011). *The real relationship in psychotherapy: The hidden foundation of change*. Washington, DC: American Psychological Association Press. http://dx.doi.org/10.1037/12349-000

Gelso, C. J., Kivlighan, D. M., Jr., & Markin, R. D. (2018). The real relationship and its role in psychotherapy outcome: A meta-analysis. *Psychotherapy*, *55*(4), 434–444. https://doi.org/10.1037/pst0000183

Greenson, R. R. (1967). *The technique and practice of psychoanalysis*. New York, NY: International Universities Press.

Kolden, G. G., Klein, M. H., Wang, C.-C., & Austin, S. B. (2011). Congruence. In J. C. Norcross (Ed.), *Psychotherapy relationships that work: Therapist contributions and responsiveness to patients* (2nd ed., pp. 187–202). New York, NY: Oxford University Press. http://dx.doi.org/10.1093/acprof:oso/9780199737208.003.0009

Kolden, G. G., Wang, C.-C., Austin, S. B., Chang, Y., & Klein, M. H. (2018). Congruence/genuineness: A meta-analysis. *Psychotherapy*, *55*(4), 424–433. https://doi.org/10.1037/pst0000162

Norcross, J. C., & Lambert, M. J. (2018). Psychotherapy relationships that work III. *Psychotherapy*, *55*(4), 303–315. http://dx.doi.org/10.1037/pst0000193

Orlinsky, D. E., Grawe, K., & Parks, B. K. (1994). Process and outcome in psychotherapy—Noch einmal. In A. E. Bergin & S. L. Garfield (Eds.), *Handbook of psychotherapy and behavior change* (4th ed., pp. 27–376). New York, NY: Wiley.

Owen, J. J., Tao, K., Leach, M. M., & Rodolfa, E. (2011). Clients' perceptions of their psychotherapists' multicultural orientation. *Psychotherapy*, *48*, 274–282. http://dx.doi.org/10.1037/a0022065

Pedersen, R. (2009). Empirical research on empathy in medicine – A critical review. *Patient Education and Counseling*, *76*, 307–322. http://dx.doi.org/10.1016/j.pec.2009.06.012

Rogers, C. R. (1957). The necessary and sufficient conditions of therapeutic personality change. *Journal of Consulting Psychology*, *21*, 95–103. http://dx.doi.org/10.1037/h0045357

Rogers, C. (1959). A theory of therapy, personality and interpersonal relationships as developed in the client-centered framework. In S. Koch (Ed.), *Psychology: A study of a science*. Vol. 3: Formulations of *the person and the social context*. New York, NY: McGraw Hill.

Truax, C. B., & Carkhuff, R. R. (1967). *Toward effective counseling and psychotherapy: Training and practice*. Chicago, IL: Aldine

Yalom, I. D. (2002). *The gift of therapy: An open letter to a new generation of therapists and their patients*. New York, NY: HarperCollins.

Chapter 8

Evidence Based Responsiveness 1: Client Factors

Daryl Mahon

Abstract

Thus far, I have introduced the reader to evidence based practice in a broad sense, and evidence based relationships across important variables. In this chapter, I further build on this by extending the need for evidence based responsiveness as applied to client factors. While the practitioner brings themselves and their bag of tools to the therapy encounter, the client brings not just their presenting problem, but their characteristic way of thinking about their problems and how they manage distress and change. Therefore, the supportive practitioner will be best served to understand how these client factors manifest for each individual that they work with. The purpose of this chapter then, is to discuss coping style, reactant level, stage of change, attachment style, and client preferences, within the context of the practitioner being responsive to these factors as they impact on therapy outcomes.

Keywords: Coping style; attachment style; reactant level; stage of change; client preference; psychotherapy variables

Chapter Learning Outcomes

(1) Examine client characteristics that impact on practitioner responsiveness.
(2) Understand the correct application of responsive interventions based on client characteristics.

Evidence Based Counselling & Psychotherapy for the 21st Century Practitioner, 85–98

Published under exclusive licence by Emerald Publishing Limited
doi:10.1108/978-1-80455-732-720231008

Introduction

Although most things a practitioner engages in can be considered to be responsive to the client, in this chapter, I have a specific meaning when speaking of responsivity. That is, evidence based responsiveness offers practitioners an empirical way to adapt the treatment style, approach, and relationship to fit trait like client characteristics. For successful outcomes to occur, practitioners must move beyond the paradigm of this treatment, for that disorder, and consider the wider context of the client. The contemporary idea of being responsive to clients can be traced back to Paul's (1967, p. 111) question: 'What treatment, by whom, is most effective for this individual with that specific problem, and under which set of circumstances?'. Unfortunately, for many, this statement has been interpreted as what set of techniques and methods can be integrated to treat a certain presenting problem. Norcross and Wampold (2018, p. 1890) critique this idea: 'perhaps the patients are diagnostically homogeneous, but nondiagnostic variability is the rule. It is precisely the unique individual and the singular context that many psychotherapists attempt to treat'. Said another way, a diagnosis may share many of the same characteristics (although this itself is questionable) for which a treatment approach might attempt to treat. However, clients with said diagnoses are vastly different in their needs based on their individual characteristics, and as such, the practitioner must adapt their treatment stance by being responsive to the client.

In this chapter, five evidence based responsive ideas are discussed: stages of change, reactance level, coping style, attachment style, and client preferences. We discuss a sixth, multicultural responsiveness in the next chapter. Critically, each of these ideas are considered to be client characteristics that the practitioner must be responsive to.

Stages of Change

As all practitioners will realise from their therapeutic work, change is a difficult process and happens differently for clients. That is, clients do not show up at our door with the same level of motivation or readiness to change. Indeed, some clients may not want to be siting with us, or in therapy at all. Clients will have different motivations, capacities for change, and readiness for change levels, influenced by their specific life experiences and worldviews. One way to help practitioners make sense of where a client is on the readiness for change trajectory, is the trans-theoretical model of change (Prochaska, DiClemente, & Velicer, 1985). This model conceptualises change as occurring over time and across five individual stages (Table 6), pre-contemplation, contemplation, preparation, action, and maintenance. In keeping with the theme of this book, this model as suggested by the name applies to all practitioners regardless of their theoretical orientation. However, what is not universal, is what clients need at different stages, and as such, it is integral that practitioners are responsive to these needs by adapting their approach, as opposed to delivering treatment protocols or modalities in isolation.

While the stages of change indicate when change happens, processes involve identifying how change happens. Change processes are the behaviours individuals

Table 6. Stages of Change Description.

Stage of Change	Description
Pre-contemplation	Clients do not intend to take action in the foreseeable future (within the next six months). Clients are often unaware that their behaviour is problematic or produces negative consequences. In this stage, the client often underestimates the pros of changing behaviour and place too much emphasis on the cons of changing behaviour
Contemplation	The client is intending to make some changes (within six months). There is some recognition that behaviour may be problematic and this is reflected in the client pro–con for change. Ambivalence can still be prevalent towards change
Preparation	There is a belief that changing behaviour is the correct thing to do. The client is ready to take action within the next 30 days
Action	Behaviour change has been initiated in the last six months with the intention to keep moving forward towards healthy behaviours. New behaviours are integrated into living life in a more healthy manner
Maintenance	The client works to prevent relapse into old unhealthy behaviours. The new behaviours have been sustained for more than six months

engage in as they attempt to acquire new healthy behaviours and modify maladaptive behaviours. Krebs, Norcross, Nicholson, and Prochaska (2018) discuss several processes of change as applied to the trans-theoretical model. For example, consciousness raising can help the client progress from pre-contemplation to contemplation, increasing awareness of the benefit of change, the effectiveness of therapy in producing change, and more insight into the presenting issue and how it manifests will be beneficial to the client. Dramatic relief is another process along the change path. Clients may mourn the loss of old behaviours or feel grief in anticipation of changing these behaviours at a future time. Self-re-evaluation is another process that occurs moving from pre-contemplation to contemplation. The client begins to think about themselves in relation to the behaviour, they assess their relationship with the problem both as it manifests, and an assessment of who they will be after the change process. As the client moves into the preparation stage, the process involved can be described as self-liberation, the client develops a belief in their ability to change unhealthy behaviours. Reinforcement is an important process, especially early on where clients will need much external reinforcement on the journey of behaviour change. However, in the action stage, clients will need to find ways of depending on their own capacity as social reinforcements may not be as plentiful. Counter-conditioning is another important process by which change is shaped. Clients develop strategies, anxieties are replaced with relaxation, negative thinking is replaced with reality checking, etc. As the client enters the maintenance stage, new alternative behaviours are being practiced, and the change process is less taxing. Stimulus control is the process by which triggers are controlled to avoid or reduce the likelihood of regression or relapsing back into the unhealthy behaviours the client previously engaged in. Summing up this process, Norcross, Krebs, and Prochaska (2011, p. 145):

> the psychotherapist's relational stance at different stages can be characterized as follows … in precontemplation, often the role is like that of a nurturing parent, who joins with a resistant and defensive youngster who is both drawn to and repelled by the prospects of becoming more independent … in contemplation, the role is akin to a Socratic teacher, who encourages clients to achieve their own insights into their condition … in the preparation stage, the stance is more like that of an experienced coach …. With clients who are progressing into action and maintenance, the psychotherapist becomes more of a consultant, who is available to provide expert advice and support when action is not progressing smoothly.

Impact of Stages of Change on Outcomes

In order to understand how the stages of change can impact on therapy outcomes and what if any moderators are relevant, we can draw on two meta-analyses. Norcross et al. (2011) illustrated that clients pre-treatment stage of change predicted outcomes with a medium effect size of d=0.46 in a sample of 32 studies with over 8,000 participants. In a second meta-analysis, Krebs et al. (2018) using a larger sample of 76 studies with 21,424 participations replicated these findings with a slightly smaller medium effect size of d=0.41. Findings tended to be consistent across treatment modality, across treatment setting, and outcome measure demonstrating robustness. However, while processes of change are found to be effective, across differential stages, matching psychotherapy type to stage of change is not supported due to lack of research in this area.

Top Tips

1. Practitioners should utilise standardised measures to assess clients' readiness for change at initial assessment.
2. Be mindful of pitfalls when working with those in pre-contemplation stage. The pros of change are often underestimated and directionality or pressure can often seem threatening. Motivational interviewing is helpful to assist the client move from pre-contemplation to contemplation.

3. Adapt the processes outlined in this chapter to the stage of change the client is in.
4. Many clients go through the cycle several times before maintenance is achieved long term. Anticipate relapse or regression to previous behaviours.
5. Practitioners should adapt a relational stance based on the stage the client is in. A nurturing parent stance with a client in pre-contemplation, a Socratic teacher role with a contemplator, an experienced coach with a client in action, and a consultant approach once into maintenance stage.

Reactance Level

Clients generally enter into therapy because they want to make some changes to their life, or how they manage their life and relationships. However, not everyone is initially motivated to enter therapy and some may feel pressurised by a significant other, or indeed a state body. Even those clients who start with gusto and energy can come up against feelings and behaviours that they do not want to face or find difficult to acknowledge and change, this is completely normal and part of the practitioner's job to work with. The term used to describe this process engaged in by a client is resistance. Many will be familiar with the idea of resistance, it goes right back to the initial work of Freud, and is proposed as a defensive mechanism. It is not surprising that many clients have an apprehension to change. However, as resistance is seen as something that generally happens within the client, practitioners tend to base their response to the client in interpretative or confrontational ways. Indeed, in many fields, resistance is seen as something for the practitioner to confront by being direct and challenging this behaviour. According to Norcross and Wampold (2018), there is a correlation between pre-contemplation stage and reactance level, which may indicate similar mechanisms underlying these processes and characteristics.

For Strong and Matross (1973), resistance emerges through the practitioners request for change, not the process of behaviour change itself. This is an important distinction for the practitioner. Another important distinction is between resistance and reactance, with the former describing resistance to change and the later describing a reactance to change. Reactance is considered as a more extreme type of resistance based on an opposition to the practitioner who is attempting to bring about change, this interpersonal reaction to the practitioner is an attempt to maintain independence and resist change (Brehm & Brehm, 1981). Beutler, Edwards, and Someah (2018, p. 1953) describe the influence of reactance on the client and how this can often manifest:

> Reactance typically decreases when the therapist avoids challenging or threatening the recipient or patient's fear of losing some

> aspect of personal freedom. And, conversely, reactance may be activated if the therapist is too confrontive or too uninvolved. The effective therapist, from this perspective, understands that any patient may directly reassert his or her freedom through oppositional behaviour within the therapy room or via premature termination.

Impact of Reactance on Outcomes

There is relatively fewer studies in this area than some of the other factors discussed in this book, however, there are two evidence syntheses of note. In their meta-analysis, Beutler et al. (2011) examined client–treatment matching applied to resistance or reactance in 12 studies with 1,102 participants. Findings suggest that clients with low levels of resistance fair better in directive therapy, while those with high levels of resistance tended to respond better to less directive therapy. This is evidenced through a large effect size of d=0.82. In an updated meta-analysis, Beutler, Kimpara et al. (2018) added another 2 studies and over 200 participants to the previous meta-analysis and had similar findings (d=0.79). Summing up the findings from this review, Beutler, Edwards, et al. (2018, p. 1960) posit that

> the results indicate that if patient reactance is not met with confrontation and control, but with acceptance and non-defensiveness, good things are more likely to happen in psychotherapy. Not quite as clearly but suggested by the linearity and strength of the findings, was the indication that the reverse is also true.

Much of these studies were conducted in Western countries with White populations, and as such drawing diversity conclusions is more difficult. However, some of the extant literature within the multicultural space would suggest that some cultures may respond more favourably to directiveness, especially where the culture has more of an authoritarian dynamic.

Top Tips

1. Assess the client's trait like reactance level, and specific in session environmental reactance if triggered.
2. Enquire as to the type of cultural background the client comes from as it relates to directiveness and authority by the practitioner.
3. Consider the modality being used, as it may be causing those with high trait like reactance to become even more reactant. Practitioners should consider therapies low in directiveness in these cases.

4. Consider the research on matching. Directive and structured therapies are more suited with low reactance clients. Becoming more of a guide and teacher at times will generally bring about better therapeutic results.
5. Consider how the collaborative approach is impacted when clients high in reactance are triggered, tend to ruptures in the alliance, and have explicit discussions about how the practitioner approach may be contributing to the client's reactance.

Coping Style

Each client brings with them to the therapy encounter a unique, yet similar way of coping with their distress. While we can consider each client to have an idiosyncratic way of coping, the research literature tends to converge in operationalising these coping styles as trait like ways of being. Much of this research emanated within the personality and social psychology realms, going back to the time of Eysenck (1947), and later on the big five factor model of Costa and McCrea (1985), which set out five main traits across domains such as introversion–extroversion among others. Not all practitioners will be familiar with trait research, but many will be familiar with the idea of internalising and externalising coping styles which are a more clinical manifestation of the introvert–extrovert spectrum (Beutler, Kimpara et al., 2018). For the responsive practitioner, adapting their approach to working with clients based on their coping style is another way of engaging in evidence based responsiveness. Coping styles are enduring personality characteristics that predispose people to manage future or current change in particular ways. It is a trait like way of behaving to mitigate distress and to adapt to situations that lie outside of one's control (Beutler & Moos, 2003).

Both internalisers and externalisers have different ways of managing distress that can become maladaptive when stress and emotionality reach levels beyond current coping capacity. Internalisers tend to be quite anxious worriers who turn into their inner worlds becoming quite self-critical and experiencing depressive states. In comparison, externalisers act out, they may blame those in their environment for their troubles. Beutler et al. (2011) provide the following analysis: Externalisers are recognisable clinically because they avoid and act out when stressed or when they face change, and they tend to blame their unhappiness and failure on the environment or others. In contrast, internalisers tend to face change and threat by the adoption of an inner blaming 'neurotic' style of coping.

Impact of Coping Style on Outcomes

With regard to previous research, there are two meta-analyses that examined psychotherapy type and coping style. Beutler et al. (2011) reviewed 12 studies and found a medium effect size of $d=0.55$ for the interaction between client coping style and therapy focus. More specifically, clients with externalising coping styles done better in symptom focussed treatment, whereas internalising styles responded more favourably to insight focussed therapy. In an updated review, Beutler, Kimpara et al. (2018) included another 6 studies in addition to the previous 12 which included almost 2,000 participants with a medium effect size of $d=0.60$ and suggested that a symptom focus proves more effective for externalising clients whereas an insight focus is generally more effective for internalisers. Given the small number of studies, most of which were conducted in the West, diversity conclusions cannot be drawn.

Top Tips

1. Assess the client's coping style through their life story and initial assessment and by enquiring into how the client manage distress.
2. Awareness of the other responsiveness characteristics such as preferences and reaction level should be considered by practitioners.
3. Practitioners will be best placed to help their externalising clients by using symptom focussed treatments such as cognitive or behavioural therapies.
4. Similarly, practitioners will find insight focussed or relationship therapies more beneficial for those with internalising coping styles.
5. Practitioners should thus acquire skills in both insight focussed/relationship therapies and cognitive and behavioural strategies in order to match clients coping style.

Attachment Style

Bowlby (1977) describes attachment as the

> propensity of human beings to make strong affectional bonds to particular others and of explaining the many forms of emotional distress and personality disturbance which unwilling separation and loss give rise to.

Early attachments are viewed as pivotal to a person developing a healthy adaptive personality and relationships with others. Ainsworth, Bell, and Stayton (1971) built on Bowlby's work developing the theory and additional attachment styles and concepts. According to Levy, Kivity, Johnson, and Gooch (2018), attachment style is a term used to describe one's characteristic way of viewing, relating to, and interacting with significant others such as parents, children, and romantic partners. Attachment styles, secure base, safe haven, and internal working models, are all concepts that the authors proposed as essential to building, maintaining, and seeking proximity to an attachment figure. There were three attachment styles initially identified by Bowlby, and a fourth later added by Ainsworth: secure, anxious-ambivalent, and avoidant. Ainsworth renamed the anxious-ambivalent pattern anxious-resistant and later identified a fourth pattern – disorganised.

As we can see these attachment styles have implications for the therapy process, and positive outcomes. It was Bowlby (1975) who distilled the main ideas of attachment as they apply to the therapy endeavour. He suggested that the aim of the practitioner is 'to provide the patient with a temporary attachment figure' (p. 191). In doing so, the practitioner provides a secure base for the client that can be utilised to explore possibilities related to present or future affectional bonds, including those with the practitioner. Bowlby (1988) describes five tasks that will be engaged in for the practitioner when working from an attachment orientated perspective:

1. The establishment of a secure base, which involves cultivating in the client a strong internal felt sense of trust and care. This safe feeling supports the client to safely explore the world, feelings, and thoughts.
2. Explore previous experiences of attachment.
3. Using the therapeutic relationship to understand relational dynamics and real-world relationships.
4. Identifying how past experiences and relationships link to the present.
5. Revising internal working models, which involve helping clients to think, behave, and feel in new ways as they relate to relationships.

It is apparent that many of these five tasks work through the therapeutic alliance. Research suggests that attachment style can change through psychotherapy as an outcome, but also attachment can be a moderator of outcomes too. Before examining the research in these areas, it is important to understand how attachment interacts with one of the main therapy variables, the therapeutic alliance. In a meta-analysis exploring the correlation between anxious attachment, avoidant attachment, and the strength of the therapeutic alliance, Bernecker, Levy, and Ellison's (2014) findings suggest that those scoring higher in both attachment styles had lower alliance scores. In a similar review, Diener and Monroe (2011) found the same correlation trajectory with regard to secure and insecure attachments and therapeutic alliance. Considering the predictive power of the alliance on outcome, tending to attachment style is important. As important, or possibly more important, is attending to alliance ruptures when they occur and the client's attachment style can impact on this too.

A more recent meta-analysis conducted by Levy et al. (2018) of 36 studies with over 3,000 participants found that clients with secure attachment styles pre-treatment, demonstrated better psychotherapy outcome (d=0.39) when compared to insecurely attached clients. As therapy progressed those who gained improvements in their attachment style may demonstrate better outcomes, while those with low pre-treatment attachment security tend to do more favourably in treatment that has an interpersonal or relational style. Younger people with avoidant attachments and older clients who are considered anxiously attached may also do worse in psychotherapy. It is important to understand that it may not be the attachment style per se that is a function of outcomes. Rather, it is possible that those who tend to be more insecurely attached can present with a host of other personality, trauma, and psychosocial factors that make therapy less successful. It is more difficult to provide diversity implications, as the authors identify 'few psychotherapy studies regularly reporting their outcome analyses as a function of age, gender, ethnicity, race, sexual orientation, or other intersecting dimensions of cultural identity' (p. 2090).

Top Tips

1. Assess client attachment style, using standardised measures, or by a structured interview format.
2. Practitioners need to be aware that attachment style will impact on outcomes, the therapeutic alliance, and how the client and practitioner relate to each other.
3. Anxiously attached clients may be difficult to treat, they may be quick to anger or feel rejected by the therapist, practitioners should consider this during interactions. Similarly, providing a structured treatment experience may be most helpful to help contain their emotional experience.
4. Practitioners should expect longer and more difficult treatment with anxiously attached clients and a quicker and more positive outcome with securely attached clients.
5. Practitioners should provide or part provide a therapy that is interpersonally/relationship focussed with those who are insecurely attached.
6. Attachment style can be modified, even in short term therapy. Practitioners should consider actively trying to modify attachment styles to secure good outcomes, indeed, it is a good outcome of itself.

Client Preferences

Shared decision making is increasingly being recognised as an effective way to deliver care and clinical interventions in routine practice. Moreover, the variety of interventions now available to support and treat different psychological and emotional distresses means that there is very often more than one treatment, or manner of delivering treatment options available to clients. Thus, assessing client's preference type is one evidence based way of improving care. Involving clients in important treatment decisions (goals, mode, style, or modality), or duration (length of treatment, number, or frequency of sessions), or who delivers treatment (gender, race, ethnicity, and sexuality) is one way that shared decision making can occur through providing preferences (Swift, Callahan, Cooper, & Parkin, 2018).

The wider research explicates that the client can have differential preference for treatment type, practitioner type, demographics such as gender, or such as cultural matching (Huey, Tilley, Jones, & Smith, 2014). Indeed, a meta-analysis found that 75% of clients preferred psychotherapy over medication within a psychiatric setting (McHugh et al., 2013). At the same time, Norcross and Wampold (2018) inform us that a client's therapy preference probably reflects in part his or her cultural values and identity. Likewise, preference is probably influenced by reactance level discussed previously, and may be an indicator of the client's coping style too. Preference accommodation is closely linked to the expectancy variables discussed in previous chapters. While outcome expectation describes what the client's belief is regarding what will happen in therapy (the outcome), client preferences speak to the client's desire for the type of therapy and experience of therapy (Swift et al., 2011). Although there are many ways to promote client preferences, Seligman (1995) suggests that the curative factor may be found in the very idea of providing choice as opposed to what specifically those choices entail.

Impact of Client Preference on Outcomes

In their meta-analysis, Lindhiem, Bennett, Trentacosta, and McLear (2014) systematically reviewed the literature examining client preferences on a host of outcomes, while using a variety of preference types. Using 34 studies, they assessed preference–outcome correlation and found the following effect sizes: with d=0.34 (treatment satisfaction), d=0.17 (treatment completion), and d=0.15 (treatment outcome). Interestingly, the authors also examined the type of preference provided to clients to establish whether differential preferences impact outcomes by type, with consistent findings in each. Summing up the findings, the authors suggest that:

> Clients who were involved in shared decision making, chose a treatment condition, or otherwise received their preferred treatment evidenced higher treatment satisfaction, increased completion rates, and superior clinical outcome, compared to clients who were not involved in shared decision making, did not choose a treatment condition, or otherwise did not receive their preferred treatment. (Lindhiem et al., 2014, p. 9)

Swift et al. (2018) replicated these findings in their meta-analysis involving 53 studies with 16,000 clients across mental health services, providing us with an effect size of d=0.28 on treatment outcomes only. Like the previous meta-analysis this review was not moderated by treatment duration, preference type, treatment options, client age, client gender, client ethnicity, or client years of education, indicating that accommodating client preferences across treatment modes, modality, treatment type, and client demographics is an evidence based practice.

This review also demonstrated that client preference was correlated with early drop out from therapy, whereby, those who did not receive their preferred treatment or choice were 1.79 times more likely to terminate early.

Top Tips

1. Where possible use a standardised or structured instrument to assess client preferences.
2. Practitioners who are trained in more than one modality should offer a choice to clients.
3. Practitioners should assess whether the client prefers the work to be more emotional, behavioural, cognitive, focussed on the past, or a mix while staying within their scope of practice.
4. Practitioners should establish early on if the client prefers who delivers the treatment (e.g. gender, race, sexuality, etc.).
5. If in a position to do so, practitioners should assess whether clients would like inpatient, community, or medication to support their treatment. This is especially important when working with a multidisciplinary team or bio-medical model.
6. Practitioners may provide choice regarding the duration of therapy, and where therapy is delivered.
7. Practitioners should ask if the client would like to utilise bibliotherapy or technology as part of the treatment process.

Conclusion

Evidence based responsivity can be achieved in the therapy endeavour by adapting the treatment approach to the client characteristics outlined in this chapter. Practitioners must be aware of, and open to the five concepts I have discussed in this chapter, as well as how some of them may interact with each other. It is clear that delivering treatment based on modalities or protocols that do not consider these characteristics will impact negatively on the therapy process. Thus, the tips provided for each characteristic should serve to help practitioners think about how they engage with such clients. In the following chapter, Ravind Jeawon and I continue the evidence based responsiveness theme by offering a whole chapter on multicultural responsiveness.

References

Ainsworth, M. D. S., Bell, S. M., & Stayton, D. J. (1971). Individual differences in strange-situation behavior of one-year-olds. In H. R. Schaffer (Ed.), *The origins of human social relations* (pp. 17–58). London: Academic Press.

Bernecker, S., Levy, K., & Ellison, W. (2014). A meta-analysis of the relation between patient adult attachment style and the working alliance. *Psychotherapy Research, 24*(1), 12–24. doi:10.1080/10503307.2013.809561

Beutler, L. E., Edwards, C., & Someah, K. (2018). Adapting psychotherapy to patient reactance level: A meta-analytic review. *Journal of Clinical Psychology*, *74*(11), 1952–1963. https://doi.org/10.1002/jclp.22682
Beutler, L. E., Harwood, T. M., Michelson, A., Song, X., & Holman, J. (2011). Resistance/reactance level. *Journal of Clinical Psychology*, *67*(2), 133–142.
Beutler, L. E., Kimpara, S., Edwards, C. J., & Miller, K. D. (2018). Fitting psychotherapy to patient coping style: A meta-analysis. *Journal of Clinical Psychology*, *74*(11), 1980–1995. https://doi.org/10.1002/jclp.22684
Beutler, L. E., & Moos, R. H. (2003). Coping and coping styles in personality and treatment planning: Introduction to the special series. *Journal of Clinical Psychology*, *59*, 1045–1048.
Bowlby, J. (1975). Attachment theory, separation anxiety and mourning. In D. A. Hamburg & K. H. Brudic (Eds.), *American handbook of psychiatry* (2nd ed., pp. 292–309). New York, NY: Basic Books.
Bowlby, J. (1977). The making and breaking of affectional bonds. I. Aetiology and psychopathology in the light of attachment theory. An expanded version of the Fiftieth Maudsley Lecture, delivered before the Royal College of Psychiatrists, 19 November 1976. *The British Journal of Psychiatry*, *130*(3), 201–210. https://doi.org/10.1192/bjp.130.3.201
Bowlby, J. (1988). Developmental psychiatry comes of age. *The American Journal of Psychiatry*, *145*(1), 1–10. https://doi.org.ezaccess.libraries.psu.edu/10.1176/ajp.145.1.1
Brehm, S. S., & Brehm, J. W. (1981). *Psychological reactance: A theory of freedom and control*. New York, NY: Academic Press.
Diener, M. J., & Monroe, J. M. (2011). The relationship between adult attachment style and therapeutic alliance in individual psychotherapy: A meta-analytic review. *Psychotherapy (Chicago, Ill.)*, *48*(3), 237–248. https://doi.org/10.1037/a0022425
Eysenck, H. J. (1947). *Dimensions of personality*. London: Routledge & Kegan Paul.
Huey, S. J., Jr, Tilley, J. L., Jones, E. O., & Smith, C. A. (2014). The contribution of cultural competence to evidence-based care for ethnically diverse populations. *Annual Review of Clinical Psychology*, *10*, 305–338. https://doi.org/10.1146/annurev-clinpsy-032813-153729
Krebs, P., Norcross, J. C., Nicholson, J. M., & Prochaska, J. O. (2018). Stages of change and psychotherapy outcomes: A review and meta-analysis. *Journal of Clinical Psychology*, *74*(11), 1964–1979. https://doi.org/10.1002/jclp.22683
Levy, K. N., Kivity, Y., Johnson, B. N., & Gooch, C. V. (2018). Adult attachment as a predictor and moderator of psychotherapy outcome: A meta-analysis. *Journal of Clinical Psychology*, *74*(11), 1996–2013. https://doi.org/10.1002/jclp.22685
Lindhiem, O., Bennett, C. B., Trentacosta, C. J., & McLear, C. (2014). Client preferences affect treatment satisfaction, completion, and clinical outcome: A meta-analysis. *Clinical Psychology Review*, *34*(6), 506–517. https://doi.org/10.1016/j.cpr.2014.06.002
McCrae, R. R., & Costa, P. T. (1985). Updating Norman's "adequacy taxonomy": Intelligence and personality dimensions in natural language and in questionnaires. *Journal of Personality and Social Psychology*, *49*(3), 710–721. https://doi.org/10.1037/0022-3514.49.3.710
McHugh, R. K., Whitton, S. W., Peckham, A. D., Welge, J. A., & Otto, M. W. (2013). Patient preference for psychological vs pharmacologic treatment of psychiatric disorders: A meta-analytic review. *The Journal of Clinical Psychiatry*, *74*(6), 595–602. https://doi.org/10.4088/JCP.12r07757
Norcross, J. C., Krebs, P. M., & Prochaska, J. O. (2011). Stages of change. *Journal of Clinical Psychology*, *67*, 143–154. https://doi.org/10.1002/jclp.20758
Norcross, J. C., & Wampold, B. E. (2018). A new therapy for each patient: Evidence-based relationships and responsiveness. *Journal of Clinical Psychology*, *74*(11), 1889–1906. https://doi.org/10.1002/jclp.22678

Prochaska, J. O., DiClemente, C. C., & Velicer, W. F. (1985). Predicting change in smoking status for self-changers. *Addictive Behaviors*, *10*(4), 395–406.
Paul, G. L. (1967). Strategy of outcome research in psychotherapy. *Journal of Consulting Psychology*, *31*(2), 109–118.
Seligman M. E. (1995). The effectiveness of psychotherapy. The consumer reports study. *The American Psychologist*, *50*(12), 965–974. https://doi.org/10.1037//0003-066x.50.12.965
Strong, S. R., & Matross, R. P. (1973). Change processes in counseling and psychotherapy. *Journal of Counseling Psychology*, *20*(1), 25–37. https://doi.org/10.1037/h0034055
Swift, J. K., Callahan, J. L., Cooper, M., & Parkin, S. R. (2018). The impact of accommodating client preference in psychotherapy: A meta-analysis. *Journal of Clinical Psychology*, *74*(11), 1924–1937. https://doi.org/10.1002/jclp.22680

Chapter 9

Evidence Based Responsiveness 2: Multicultural Considerations

Ravind Jeawon and Daryl Mahon

Abstract

In this chapter, Ravind Jeawon and I discuss the ideas around being responsive to diversity in an evidence based manner. Although this chapter belongs within the evidence based responsiveness section discussed in the previous chapter, we both considered it essential to provide a whole chapter on its theory and application, as it is an integral area often overlooked in clinical training and provided a curtesy overview during ongoing professional development and clinical supervision. The multicultural literature uses different terminology to refer to the practice of responsiveness, we discuss these ideas and the evidence base for them, while introducing the reader to other processes and theories which will help developing practitioners make sense of what can be a vastly complex area of clinical work. Several adapted, real life case examples are drawn from Ravind's clinical experience to encourage reflection and provide insight into these processes.

Keywords: Multicultural competency; multicultural orientation; cultural humility; intersectionality; microaggression; diversity and inclusion

Chapter Learning Outcomes

(1) Appreciate the various components of multicultural responsive therapy.
(2) Identify how best to apply these practice to your specific context.

Evidence Based Counselling & Psychotherapy for the 21st Century Practitioner, 99–114

Published under exclusive licence by Emerald Publishing Limited
doi:10.1108/978-1-80455-732-720231009

Introduction

Multicultural responsiveness when delivering treatment and providing effective care has been topical for at least five decades. The formation of the Association of Black Psychologists in the United States in 1968 foreshadowed the beginnings of a multicultural competency movement that impacted psychology, psychiatry, and social care disciplines in the coming decades. The contemporary discourse around evidence based practice provides an opportunity to revisit this area, often described as the fourth force in psychotherapy while also addressing potential limitations. Multicultural identities are a multidimensional construct informed by an individual's gender, age, religion, ethnicity, race, socioeconomic status, sexual orientation, national origin, heritage, and disability status. Cultural identity is a complex, dynamic construct consisting of various aspects of an individual or group of individuals.

According to Mahon and Jeawon (2022), cultural responsiveness is the process by which individuals and systems respond respectfully and effectively to the diversity within individuals from all cultural backgrounds, embracing differences across language, gender, religion, spiritual tradition, and socioeconomic or ethnic backgrounds, alongside other aspects of cultural richness. Much of the extant literature speaks about this way of working using competency terminology. However, both authors view the competency terminology to be problematic, as do other researchers within the field (Davis et al., 2018; Owen et al., 2016). The rationale for this critique is based on the vast intersectional, multicultural identities that often present within those who come for therapy and the dynamic nature of the construct of culture itself. This makes the task of competency almost impossible for the average practitioner working within diversity in routine practice and the idea of being 'competent' with a set of specific, measurable, and clinical skills implausible as a general method of working. This fact is underscored by outcomes research which indicates competencies in general psychotherapy account for a mere 1% of the variance in outcome (Wampold & Imel, 2015).

Multicultural Competency

Notwithstanding these issues, the multicultural competency literature continues to offer concepts and ideas that are helpful. One of the most recognised models of cultural competency is the person-based model (Chu, Leino, Pflum, & Sue, 2016). This model proposes three components: self-awareness of one's own cultural background and how this impacts practice; knowledge about the worldview, values, and culture of those from diverse cultural backgrounds; and learning skills in culturally appropriate treatment interventions (Sue, Arredondo, & McDavis, 1992). Sometimes called the tripartite model (Chu et al., 2016), the person-based model continues to influence design and implementation of cultural competency training alongside professional examination in psychotherapy to this day. This chapter will examine this area in more detail, flagging some risk trainers' and practitioners' face attempting to be culturally competent. An over focus on competency can lead to concentration on specific areas of the tripartite model, running the risk of generalising or re-stereotyping clients which poses a significant risk to the working alliance. To mitigate against this sort of risk, the chapter explores a series of individual but interconnected concepts which need careful consideration when describing how practitioners can become responsive to diverse multicultural identities in the therapeutic environment. This is presented as an evolution of the existing multicultural competency literature in the spirit of evidence based practice.

The multicultural competency (MCC) approach stipulates three broad ideas:

- That there are a set of competencies that can impact client outcomes and can be acquired by therapists through a standardised training regime.
- Competency in these skills can be assessed and identified in the therapist.
- The competencies are a standard characteristic across client populations.

Clinical Example

Before further discussion on cultural responsiveness let's pause to look at a brief example based on a real clinical situation from a service known for its efforts towards cultural competency. This adapted example was shared as part of a discussion exploring early dropout from certain services by African born clients.

> Santu had been seeking asylum for three months and concerned for her welfare support workers had referred her to a specialist counselling service with expertise supporting survivors of traumatic events using culturally competent care. Santu spoke Lingala and this required an interpreter to assist in the sessions. After three sessions, Santu broke down laughing telling the interpreter that this was 'a ridiculous process' and that there was no point continuing as it 'wasn't helpful', she did however feedback that her chats with the interpreter before sessions and even during sessions had been helpful and that she would miss them.

The example is short and has a few threads to it, a triad is in place when working with an interpreter which poses certain challenges but was a necessary cultural adaption to the provision of counselling in this instance. As we discuss the topic of being multiculturally responsive through the lens of evidence based practice we invite the reader to reflect on this example and consider the following:

(a) What is going on in this example in terms of the provision of effective care?
(b) What might have led to the process being described as 'ridiculous'?
(c) What if anything might have been more helpful?
(d) Why was this information not captured?
(e) Which of the common factors may be relevant here?

Cultural Adaptations Research

Cultural adaptations are one way that practitioners can become responsive to the multicultural identity of clients to help improve outcomes. Several domains that can be culturally adapted are cited by Bernal, Bonilla, and Bellido (1995) and include language, persons, metaphors, content, concepts, goals, methods, and context. It has been noted in the previous chapters that those with diverse, minoritised identities are not represented within trials testing evidence based therapies (Huey, Tilley, Jones, & Smith, 2014; Sue et al., 2013). At the same time, research indicates that some practitioners demonstrate better outcomes with clients who identify as white than those of diverse ethnicity (Drinane, Owen, & Kopta, 2016; Hayes, Owen, & Bieschke, 2015; Imel et al., 2011). What we do know, is that broadly speaking being culturally responsive has demonstrated across several meta-analyses and evidence syntheses to be an effective method of improving outcomes for culturally diverse populations (Benish, Quintana, & Wampold, 2011; Davis et al., 2018; Griner & Smith, 2006; Smith, Rodríguez, & Bernal, 2011; Soto, Smith, Griner, Domenech Rodríguez, & Bernal, 2018; Tao et al., 2018). Smith et al. (2011) in a meta-analysis of 65 studies found that culturally adopted treatments had a medium effect size of d=0.46, with treatments adopting symbols and metaphors that match the client's cultural worldview and treatments to specific monocultural identities being more effective. Griner and Smith's (2006) meta-analysis found that treatment adapted to specific cultural identities was as much as four times as effective compared against non-adapted, and matching clients to therapists who speak their own language were up to twice as effective.

Benish et al. (2011) found that culturally adapted psychotherapy for race/ethnicity is more effective than un-adapted compared against bona fide therapies. Adapting treatment to meet the client's explanatory health model with regard to beliefs about distress, onset, manifestation, and treatment options within the cultural understanding of the client is thought to be the main mechanism of change. Tao, Owen, Pace, and Imel's (2018) meta-analysis suggest that client ratings of practitioners' multicultural competency accounts for approximately 37% of the variance in the therapeutic alliance and 52% of the variance in client satisfaction. Accordingly, therapist's multicultural competency can be considered an important empirically supported therapeutic relational factor, with a variance of approximately 8.4% on outcomes.

Some Notable Cultural Adaptations

As stated previously, making cultural adaptations to fit specific demographics can be helpful, and while the list of adaptations to fit differential cultural characteristics is far from exhaustive, the three areas below are likely to be more transtheoretical and prevalent in routine practice and are discussed very briefly.

Religion/Spirituality

Many clients who experience religion or spirituality as a salient part of their identity would like the practitioner to integrate these beliefs and values within psychotherapy (Vieten et al., 2013). In fact, my colleague Dr Jeb Brown, whose chapter you will read from in the next section of the book, conducted a study into the relationship between spiritual struggles and mental health. This study with 1,800 participants demonstrated that across the course of therapy, as spiritual struggles decreased so too did mental health distress (Harris, et al., 2016). This implies that practitioners who can attend to this cultural adaptation will have clients who do better in therapy. Indeed, in their meta-analyses of 100 studies and almost 8,000 participants, Captari et al. (2018) demonstrated that adapting therapy to the client's spiritual values and beliefs predicted better outcomes across psychological and spiritual measures.

LGBTQ+

While religion and spirituality are complex identity factors, so too is sexuality and it needs to be considered also. Affirmative psychotherapy highlights the unequal power inherent in the client–practitioner relationship, which may prove more pronounced in those relationships involving those with minoritised sexual identities and heterosexual practitioners. Thus, the responsibility of providing responsive methods rests with the practitioner, not the client (Moradi & Budge, 2018). Moreover, we must not assume that those with similar sexualities are a homogenous group, diversity within diversity is the rule not the exception:

> LGBQ+ identities are diverse, culturally situated, and dynamic, as reflected in the expanding inclusivity of sexual identity labels (e.g., L, G, B, Q). Moreover, LGBQ+ people as a group represent all ages, classes, genders, ethnicities, races, and other sociodemographic characteristics. Acknowledging this diversity among LGBQ+ populations is critical. (p. 2037)

As such, individualisation of knowledge about sexually diverse people is congruent with an 'informed not-knowing stance' (Laird, 2000). That is, the practitioner expresses genuine curiosity to try understanding the client and their identity more deeply, rather than assume a pre-conceived textbook understanding. We come back to this idea when we discuss cultural humility later in the chapter. As an emerging area of interest, LGBTQ+ and gender, discussed below, do not have as much of a research base as other concepts discussed in this chapter, or book; yet they are of real importance too.

Gender

Gender is defined by systems of power that shape and are shaped by gender norms and hierarchies that intersect with other systems of power such as race, sexual orientation, and class. These norms and hierarchies disadvantage transgender people relative to cisgender people and disadvantage women relative to men (Budge & Moradi, 2018, p. 2015). It is important for the practitioner not to overemphasise gender, while at the same time not to underemphasis it. In addition, it is essential to privilege the clients experience and identify how gender interacts with other important identity characteristics, through intersectionality. This later point is important, while much of the adaptations discussed so far have been described for specific demographics (ethnocultural adaptations) the reality is that individuals attend therapy with multiple identities, and the average practitioner will generally work with people with various multicultural identities. Therefore, general principles and processes may be the most efficient and effective way for practitioners to be responsive to a wider population of people and their intersectional identities.

Intersectionality

Psychotherapy does not exist in a vacuum and power and privilege are present to some degree in the therapeutic relationship even before the first session has occurred. Like many disciplines, psychotherapy is entrenched in its own history; theories and models often formulated by western practitioners with individualistic cultural outlooks, immersed in the attitudes, prejudices, and language of their eras. As practitioners we are culturally encapsulated by our lived experience, clinical experience, core training, and modality preferences which may pose difficulty when providing culturally responsive care. We have already noted that psychotherapy research is not immune from the area of bias often designed around specific populations of clients. The past 40 years may have introduced exciting new models and protocols, but modern research indicates very little in terms of improved client outcomes.

Intersectionality is a theoretical framework for understanding how aspects of a person's social and political identities combine to create different modes of discrimination and privilege. For example, gender, caste, sex, race, class, sexuality, religion, disability, and physical appearance (Crenshaw, 1993). Clients and practitioners are likely to have multiple cultural identities that intersect giving differing experiences of privilege or oppression that may be pertinent to their lived experience. This is important to consider when being culturally responsive to traditional presenting issues such as anxiety, depression, or relationship problems and affords the opportunity of enhancing crucial pan-theoretical factors essential for effective outcomes in therapy such as empathy, managing transference, and positive regard/affirmation augmenting the overall working alliance.

As such, it is important for practitioners not to make assumptions about any one aspect of a client's identity, but rather to be open to how different aspects may intersect and become more prominent in the therapeutic encounter. Most practitioners will contend that being open, curious, and non-judgemental are instrumental to all therapeutic encounters but research on *microaggression* in sessions (discussed later) gives us a hint that from a multicultural perspective practitioner awareness of power, privilege, and how culturally encapsulated they are may be a bigger block to successful outcomes than they appreciate. For example, *within* group differences can often be more pronounced than *between* group differences. Take two individuals identifying as the same race, the intersection of sexuality, socioeconomic status, or gender can provide for very different experiences of racial identity which could also play out in the therapeutic encounter.

As such, intersectionality provides the practitioner with a theoretical framework and awareness of how different intersecting identities may impact the client's experience. Viewed through this lens, it becomes quite apparent how the language of cultural competency can be limiting our understanding of these issues within the therapeutic process. Our own privilege or lack thereof alongside our own culturally encapsulated existence provides notable obstacles in understanding others, both in terms of clinical practice and the type of research we conduct. It is thus a significant issue when considering the common factors from a multicultural perspective. The very fact that a vulnerable person in distress is being referred for or is paying to sit with a specialist sets up a dynamic that can be particularly challenging for individuals minoritised outside the therapy room. The risk here is that well intentioned practitioners may unintentionally repeat or reinforce problematic dynamics present for clients in their day to day lives within the therapeutic setting. Culturally responsive practitioners are aware of this and can address these issues with clients collaboratively using the working alliance. Culturally blind practitioners tend to ignore these issues (even when they are made explicit by clients) and may face issues like problematic enactments in sessions leading to early dropout as was the case in with Santu. Cultural humility (discussed later in multicultural orientation, MCO) is one method that can help support practitioners to become more responsive to cultural differences.

Clinical Example

> An ethnically minoritized therapist built a good relationship over two years with a white client accessing low-cost counselling and was attempting to solicit feedback. When doing so he noticed the client repeatedly commented on being surprised about having had a positive experience with a male therapist, sharing that initially they had serious reservations about working with him. This was explored as very positive feedback in supervision. The client left therapy suddenly shortly after this session with no explanation.

If we revisit this example from a culturally responsive viewpoint, this positive conclusion may be premature. From the perspective of intersectionality an opportunity emerged here to take the client's lead and explore difference. Gender was mentioned but ethnicity, sexuality, socio economic status, and other variables like age may all be relevant too. The practitioner felt happy receiving positive feedback and maintained comfort, potentially missing the opportunity to 'lean in' both in session and in supervision to fully explore what might be going on. Difference and silence were presenting issues for this client and within the relationship cultural silence may have fed an enactment limiting how far the alliance could go.

Microaggression

Microaggression is a term used for brief and commonplace daily verbal or behavioural indignities, whether intentional or unintentional, that communicate hostile, derogatory, or negative attitudes towards stigmatised or culturally marginalised groups (Sue & Sue, 2016). It is important for practitioners to differentiate between the general everyday rudeness/impoliteness all people may experience and microaggression. Microaggressions send denigrating messages to individuals because of their group membership (e.g. race, gender, culture, religion, social class, sexual orientation, etc.). The effects of microaggression are constant, cumulative, and often last the lifespan of an individual, family, or community. It's impact and presence when named is often dismissed as being oversensitive or overreacting, particularly by those in a position of privilege. Subtle racism, elitism, sexism, and heterosexism can remain relatively invisible and potentially harmful to the wellbeing, self-esteem, and standard of living of many groups in society. These common daily, experiences leave many people feeling vulnerable, targeted, angry, and afraid. As such, those who have experienced microaggression suffer psychological distress, including an increase in symptoms of depression, anxiety, and post-traumatic stress disorder, and can face backlash if they speak up (Abdullah et al., 2021; Torres & Taknint, 2015).

Clinical Example

> Adellah was referred for counselling by the student support service of her university. She was looking for help with sleep issues also describing chronic pain and feelings of depression and hopelessness, impacting her postgraduate studies. Her background was from a minority sect in India where she had been a top student and worked professionally for some time before pursuing further studies. She had completed a Masters abroad which she described as a positive experience but since starting a PHD programme in a new university things had got markedly worse.
>
> Adellah found counselling helpful initially and described a good relationship forming over six months of weekly therapy. The most recent two months of therapy with this practitioner were difficult and the client was beginning to feel worse. She reported her mood and physical health were declining and brought to therapy recent experiences as a 'woman of colour' – this was repeatedly met with responses like, 'I see only a woman, not a woman of colour'. The inability to bring this part of herself to an otherwise good relationship eventually frustrated the client so much so she left her therapist to look for a different practitioner.

The microaggression in question here is described by Sue and Sue (2016) as *Colour Blindness*, namely the belief that race/ethnicity is not important and subsequently not considered. Attitudes like 'There is only one race, the human race', or 'we are all the same under our skin' would be other examples of colour-blindness. It is possible that well intentioned practitioners do not recognise racial–ethnic microaggressions when they occur or feel anxiety about the process of addressing them, which of course means that an alliance rupture will fail to be repaired.

In several studies of white and ethnically diverse practitioners, the demonstration of *colour-blind* attitudes in session was evident but associated with a practitioner's genuine compassionate and empathic belief. This means that practitioners attempting to do a good job and use empathy may introduce a microaggression that invalidates a person's experience and multicultural identity by inferring an individual assimilate to the dominant culture (Sue & Sue, 2016). It also risks dissolving cultural opportunities as they emerge in sessions something we will discuss later. Across other aspects of cultural identity, such as gender, socio economic status, sexuality, disability, or religion this could be termed *culture blindness*. The concern here is that the therapeutic process could become an environment rife with microaggression. High rates of racial–ethnic microaggressions are reported by those seeking support services. Hook et al. (2016) highlight that between 53% and 81% of clients accessing supports reported at least one microaggression. Owen et al. (2018) found that clients' who experienced microaggressions from their practitioner experience worse therapeutic alliances and worse therapy outcomes. At the same time, Owen et al (2018) found that practitioners' ability to identify one of three microaggressions in simulated sessions was between 38% and 52%. Clients who perceive racial–ethnic microaggressions from their practitioner have reported lower satisfaction in the relationship and poorer outcomes, demonstrating it is integral for any multiculturally responsive practitioner to identify and limit microaggressions and their potential to re-traumatise individuals in therapeutic settings.

Multicultural Orientation

Earlier in the chapter, we challenged the idea that more competency-based training holds the answers to issues that limit the provision of effective culturally responsive care. Consideration of an evidence based approach, the MCO which consists of three interconnected and interdependent ideas: *cultural humility*, *cultural opportunity*, and *cultural comfort* (Table 7), may be of more use for therapists working with diverse caseloads. The orientation approach is more aligned to a process and attitude on the part of the practitioner, not a competency that can be taught through a protocol with fidelity. It is a pan-theoretical approach that practitioners can use to be responsive to diverse multicultural populations' including issues discussed above such as intersectionality and microaggression. For Watkins et al. (2019), the MCO can be viewed 'as a process-oriented, attitudes-additive perspective to the existing MCC Knowledge Skills and Attitude (KSA) competency framework'.

How practitioners use the MCO will be influenced by many factors such as the values and worldview they hold, experiential avoidance, and their awareness of other cultural dynamics. Davis et al. (2018) describe this process as a cultural

Table 7. MCO Framework.

Cultural humility	Being aware of cultural and power dynamics that are at play between therapist and the client and approaching these issues without defensiveness but with collaboration (Hook et al., 2016)
Cultural opportunities	Cultural opportunities are 'markers that occur in therapy in which the client's cultural beliefs, values or other aspects of the client's cultural identity could be explored' (Owen et al., 2016). They occur when clients' mention their beliefs, values, or other details that provide an opportunity for the therapist to explore the client's cultural identities in more depth
Cultural comfort	Cultural comfort is characterised by feeling at ease, open, calm, or relaxed with diversity (Davis et al., 2018). As such, cultural comfort refers to the therapist's thoughts and feelings that emerge before, during, and after conversations about the client's cultural identities or culturally focussed content

enactment entailing worldviews, values, and beliefs of both the client and therapist interacting and influencing one another to cocreate a relational experience in the spirit of healing. As such, one practitioner's response may look entirely different than another. The following three components of MCO will provide the practitioner with a framework to help guide their practice.

Cultural humility can be considered the bedrock of the MCO approach. Increasingly, those across disciplines within the mental health domains have come to understand humility as an alternative to, and/or complementary language to the competency approach (Davies et al., 2018; Foronda et al., 2016).

Humility is conceptualised as consisting of both intrapersonal and interpersonal components.

- A level of self-awareness regarding the view a practitioner holds of themselves, and their limitations.
- The extent to which a practitioner can hold an interpersonal position with a client that is curious about their client's cultural identity.
- A stance that does not assume one knows what meaning is ascribed to such cultural identities.

Hook et al. (2016) demonstrated that for clients' who experienced microaggressions in session, cultural humility predicted the number and impact of these aggressions after controlling for general multicultural competencies, indicating the added value of cultural humility. While cultural humility may be the foundation to this orientation, Watkins et al. (2019) suggest that on its own, it may not be enough to improve outcomes. If cultural humility is the motivational factor for practitioners who want to find out about others important identities, then *cultural opportunity and cultural comfort* can be considered the in-session components where potential cultural markers are identified and broached. Said another way, through cultural humility, practitioners identify important cultural markers as they present in session and broach the subject using cultural opportunities. Owen et al. (2016) describe cultural opportunities as those points in a session where important cultural beliefs, values, and identities are present and can be explored by both practitioner and client. The clinical examples above all represent cultural opportunities. Therapists should feel that they can broach these issues if judged to be of therapeutic value in situations where cultural opportunities may not be manifest or explicit. Davies et al. (2018) suggest doing this gently and authentically and without big transitions or forcing the issue.

Hence, practitioners who practice cultural humility and opportunity will have a certain level of ease with engaging in these practices, that is, cultural comfort. Cultural comfort explains the level of ease that practitioners' experience before, during, and after conversations with clients about their cultural identities (Owen et al., 2017). While cultural comfort would be needed to navigate the complex interpersonal dynamics that occur in session, cultural discomfort may be a good indication that something has been triggered and needs attending to. The earlier examples of Adellah (and potentially Santu) suggest practitioner discomfort which led to the colour blind microaggression in session. Davies et al. (2018) use the language of cultural transference and counter-transference to describe these dynamics and viewed through this lens, feelings of cultural discomfort may precede cultural humility and would seem important for practitioners to identify as they may impede therapeutic progress.

The evidence for MCO in therapy is emerging as strong across a number of studies (Davies et al., 2018; Hook, Davis, Owen, Worthington, & Utsey, 2013; Hook et al., 2016; Owen et al., 2014, 2016). In a retrospective study, Owen et al. (2016) examined therapist cultural humility and missed opportunities. Findings suggest that clients' who rated their therapist as culturally humble had better therapy outcomes, while those who rated their therapist as having missed opportunities to discuss their cultural identity (cultural opportunity) reported worse outcomes. Again, Owen et al. (2014) in a study focussed on religious cultural identities reported that therapists who were more culturally humble with religious clients' had better outcomes. This suggests that working with a MCO seems to be mediated by the overall therapeutic alliance. Hook et al. (2013) found that cultural humility was correlated with the alliance and also demonstrated that cultural humility correlated with the alliance and client outcomes found that cultural humility mediates the alliance and client outcomes.

Multicultural Alliance Rupture–Repair

You will recall that in the evidence based relationships chapter, the idea of alliance rupture–repair was introduced. This concept holds as much, if not more, within a multicultural context. You will remember from our earlier discussion on microaggressions how easily these can happen when the practitioner is unaware of such processes, and the negative impact that these can have on outcomes, and the therapeutic alliance, through ruptures (Hook et al., 2013; Owen et al., 2016). One method to help practitioners' identity and repair ruptures is using feedback (previous chapters). This is discussed, albeit implicitly at times in the multicultural literature, however, methods to do this are not provided. For example, Soto et al. (2018) suggest that:

> client ratings of therapist multicultural competencies strongly predict their engagement and outcomes in treatment. Notably, this finding held only for client ratings, so clients' perceptions of the therapist are consequential and can be solicited by therapists.

However, they fail to suggest what strategies can be utilised to achieve this. With regard to addressing racial microaggressions that have negatively impacted on the alliance, Yeo and Torres-Harding (2021) found that clients had improved alliances when the practitioner engaged in rupture–repair strategies. Using feedback-informed care is proposed here as a way to address multicultural alliance ruptures, the process for doing this is the same as the protocols and processes discussed previously.

Top Tips

(1) Multicultural responsiveness is something for *all* practitioners to consider within their individual practice. It is not a 'competency' to be left to specialised services or trainings. Its impact on evidence based variables important for client outcomes like the collaborative working alliance and empathy may be crucial for certain clients. Its consideration is also relevant with other important evidence based variables like client preference accommodation or cultural adaptions to therapeutic work.

(2) We are all culturally rich beings, it is linked to our identities, we have had experiences that allow us describe aspects of ourselves such as where we come from, our family of origin, what age we consider ourselves to be, our sexual identity, religion, or even physical appearance. It is not an area just linked to race and ethnicity even though these may be very relevant too.

(3) With point two in mind consider the impact of intersectionality, power, privilege, and oppression – could it be present at all when delivering care, making assessments, referrals, or your own hypothesis? Could it be relevant to your caseload, to early dropout or therapeutic ruptures/transference?

(4) Also consider your own beliefs, attitudes, politics, and opinions – could any of this impact demonstrating cultural humility in sessions when responding to difference.

(5) Embrace the spirit of cultural comfort and opportunity. There is permission here to lean into cultural material if relevant in sessions – microaggression, difficulty with pronouns, assumptions around physical health, or disability if caught all provide cultural opportunity. If unattended to, these may lead to early dropout and a variety of other negative outcomes. Collaborate around potential mistakes or ruptures when they occur, this can really strengthen the alliance and also provide real validation and healing that may not be occurring outside the counselling room.
(6) Some of the above advice is general and may be hard to judge when in session or later in supervision, particularly with a varied client caseload. Practitioner cultural discomfort, ruptures, or challenges with certain clients can be very nuanced especially when code switching or 'passing' is a phenomenon with minoritised individuals. To attend to this consistently, reflect on how you collaboratively solicit structured feedback in each session. This can really guide difficult work and enhance when a response is needed.
(7) Responding to difference has to be considered within in the laws of your jurisdiction and also the ethical context of organisations you represent and your own ethics personally. Some issues that have cultural overtones can be particularly challenging and may require additional support or communication with other agencies. Requests for conversion therapy or a tolerance for content like hebephilia, female genital mutilation, rape, or abusive parenting can all pose significant ethical and legal challenges. There are limits to how much we can lean in and as practitioners we need to be honest and kind with ourselves around this.

Conclusion

Delivering training and presentations around multicultural responsiveness in recent years has made both authors aware of a multitude of diverse reactions and feelings among practitioners and organisations. Fear and discomfort are perhaps to be expected but a sense of loss is another feeling often expressed. The area can be overwhelming and unsettling if not handled with care. Shaming and silencing practitioners is not collaborative or helpful, potentially echoing polarising discussions and 'cancel culture' type dynamics running broadly through the external environment therapy is located within. Anand and Winters (2008) suggest that some of the unintended consequences of diversity and unconscious bias trainings can be leaving people feeling confused, angry, and with even more animosity towards difference. The multicultural responsiveness approach discussed above promotes listening rather than lecturing and leaning into difference rather than away. Practitioner's reflection on cultural adaptions to how we work or indeed when we decide to refer are important. The presence of power dynamics and privilege within sessions (and clinical supervision) are also acknowledged through intersectionality. Acknowledgement of privilege can sound negative to some as can naming oppression, but the therapeutic environment provides wonderful opportunity for healing and validation in this area, potentially impossible externally for reasons that are neither the practitioner nor client's fault. Mistakes will happen and there needs to be permission for this but also a way to address and remedy them. The MCO provides a way to view responding to difference that tones down some of the high-stakes language around competency. There is permission to address issues like microaggression, unconscious bias, and misattuned empathy through alliance rupture–repair and an opportunity to integrate client feedback no matter what modality is being used. We may never know for sure what was behind Santu's laugh earlier but incorporating the topics discussed throughout this chapter into our individual professional identity should give us a greater chance of understanding next time.

References

Abdullah, T., Graham-LoPresti, J. R., Tahirkheli, N. N., Hughley, S. M., & Watson, L. T. J. (2021). Microaggressions and posttraumatic stress disorder symptom scores among Black Americans: Exploring the link. *Traumatology*, *27*(3), 244–253. https://doi.org/10.1037/trm0000259

Anand, R., & Winters, M. F. (2008). A retrospective view of corporate diversity training from 1964 to the present. *Academy of Management Learning & Education*, *7*(3), 356–372.

Benish, S. G., Quintana, S., & Wampold, B. E. (2011). Culturally adapted psychotherapy and the legitimacy of myth: A direct-comparison meta-analysis. *Journal of Counseling Psychology*, *58*(3), 279–289. https://doi.org/10.1037/a0023626

Bernal, G., Bonilla, J., & Bellido, C. (1995). Ecological validity and cultural sensitivity for outcome research: Issues for the cultural adaptation and development of psychosocial treatments with Hispanics. *Journal of Abnormal Child Psychology*, *23*(1), 67–82.

Budge, S. L., & Moradi, B. (2018). Attending to gender in psychotherapy: Understanding and incorporating systems of power. *Journal of Clinical Psychology*, *74*(11), 2014–2027. https://doi.org/10.1002/jclp.22686

Captari, L. E., Hook, J. N., Hoyt, W., Davis, D. E., McElroy-Heltzel, S. E., & Worthington, E. L., Jr. (2018). Integrating clients' religion and spirituality within psychotherapy: A comprehensive meta-analysis. *Journal of Clinical Psychology*, *74*(11), 1938–1951. https://doi.org/10.1002/jclp.22681

Chu, J., Leino, A., Pflum, S., & Sue, S. (2016). A model for the theoretical basis of cultural competency to guide psychotherapy. *Professional Psychology: Research and Practice*, *47*, 18–29.

Crenshaw, K. (1993). Mapping the margins: Intersectionality, identity politics, and violence against women of color. *Stanford Law Review*, *43*(6), 1241–1279.

Davis, D. E., DeBlaere, C., Owen, J., Hook, J. N., Rivera, D. P., Choe, E., & Placeres, V. (2018). The multicultural orientation framework: A narrative review. *Psychotherapy*, *55*(1), 89–100. http://dx.doi.org/10.1037/pst0000160

Drinane, J. M., Owen, J., & Kopta, M. (2016). Racial/ethnic disparities in psychotherapy: Does the outcome matter? *Testing, Psychometrics, Methodology in Applied Psychology*, *23*, 531–544.

Foronda, C., MacWilliams, B., & McArthur, E. (2016). Interprofessional communication in healthcare: An integrative review. *Nurse Education in Practice*, *19*, 36–40. https://doi.org/10.1016/j.nepr.2016.04.005

Griner, D., & Smith, T. B. (2006). Culturally adapted mental health intervention: A meta-analytic review. *Psychotherapy: Theory, Research, Practice, Training*, *43*(4), 531–548. https://doi.org/10.1037/0033-3204.43.4.531

Harris, N., Pargament, K., Sisemore, T., & Brown, J. (2016). The relationship of decline in spiritual struggles to psychotherapy outcomes: Evidence from a large scale survey of psychotherapy clients. *Christian Psychology*.

Hayes, J. A., Owen, J., & Bieschke, K. J. (2015). Therapist differences in symptom change with racial/ethnic minority clients. *Psychotherapy*, *52*, 308–314. http://dx.doi.org/10.1037/a0037957

Hook, J. N., Davis, D. E., Owen, J., Worthington, E. L., Jr, & Utsey, S. O. (2013). Cultural humility: Measuring openness to culturally diverse clients. *Journal of Counseling Psychology*, *60*, 353–366. http://dx.doi.org/10.1037/a0032595

Hook, J. N., Farrell, J. E., Davis, D. E., DeBlaere, C., Van Tongeren, D. R., & Utsey, S. O. (2016). Cultural humility and racial microaggressions in counseling. *Journal of Counseling Psychology*, *63*, 269–277. http://dx.doi.org/10.1037/cou0000114

Huey, S. J., Jr, Tilley, J. L., Jones, E. O., & Smith, C. A. (2014). The contribution of cultural competence to evidence-based care for ethnically diverse populations. *Annual Review of Clinical Psychology*, *10*, 305–338. https://doi.org/10.1146/annurev-clinpsy-032813-153729

Imel, Z. E., Baldwin, S., Atkins, D. C., Owen, J., Baardseth, T., & Wampold, B. E. (2011). Racial/ethnic disparities in therapist effectiveness: A conceptualization and initial study of cultural competence. *Journal of Counseling Psychology*, *58*, 290–298. http://dx.doi.org/10.1037/a0023284

Laird, J. (2000). Theorizing culture: Narrative ideas and practice principles. *Journal of Feminist Family Therapy*, *11*, 99–114 https://doi.org/10.1300/J086v11n04_08

Mahon, D., & Jeawon, R. (2022). Diverse, intersecting and multicultural considerations in trauma-responsive organisations. *Trauma-responsive organisations: The trauma ecology model* (pp. 91–108). Bingley: Emerald Publishing Limited. https://doi.org/10.1108/978-1-80382-429-120221006

Moradi, B., & Budge, S. L. (2018). Engaging in LGBQ+ affirmative psychotherapies with all clients: Defining themes and practices. *Journal of Clinical Psychology*, *74*(11), 2028–2042. https://doi.org/10.1002/jclp.22687

Owen, J., Drinane, J., Tao, K. W., Adelson, J. L., Hook, J. N., Davis, D. & Fookune N. (2017). Racial/ethnic disparities in client unilateral termination: The role of therapists' cultural comfort. *Psychotherapy Research*, *27*(1), 102–111. doi:10.1080/10503307.2015.1078517

Owen, J., Jordan, T., Turner, D., Davis, D., Hook, J., & Leach, M. (2014). Therapists' multicultural orientation: Cultural humility, spiritual/religious identity, and therapy outcomes. *Journal of Psychology and Theology*, *42*, 91–99.

Owen, J., Tao, K. W., & Drinane, J. M. (2018). Microaggressions: Clinical impacts and psychological harm. In C. M. Capodilupo, K. L. Nadal, D. P. Rivera, D. W. Sue, & G. C. Torino (Eds.), *Microaggression theory: Influence and implications* (pp. 67–85). New York, NY: John Wiley & Sons.

Owen, J., Tao, K. W., Drinane, J. M., Hook, J. N., Davis, D. E., & Kune, N. F. (2016). Client perceptions of therapists' multicultural orientation: Cultural (missed) opportunities and cultural humility. *Professional Psychology: Research and Practice*, *47*, 30–37. http://dx.doi.org/10.1037/pro0000046

Smith, T. B., Rodríguez, M. D., & Bernal, G. (2011). Culture. *Journal of Clinical Psychology*, *67*, 166–175. https://doi.org/10.1002/jclp.20757

Soto, A., Smith, T. B., Griner, D., Domenech Rodríguez, M., & Bernal, G. (2018). Cultural adaptations and therapist multicultural competence: Two meta-analytic reviews. *Journal of Clinical Psychology*, *74*(11), 1907–1923. https://doi.org/10.1002/jclp.22679

Sue, S. (2006). Cultural competency: From philosophy to research and practice. *Journal of Community Psychology*, *34*, 237–245. https://doi.org/10.1002/jcop.20095

Sue, D. W., Arredondo, P., & McDavis R. J. (1992). Multicultural counseling competencies and standards: A call to the profession. *Journal of Counseling & Development*, *70*, 477–486. https://doi.org/10.1002/j.1556-6676.1992.tb01642.x

Sue, D. W., & Sue, S. (2016). *Counseling the culturally diverse: Theory and practice* (7th ed.). Hoboken, NJ: John Wiley.

Tao, K. W., Owen, J., Pace, B. T., & Imel, Z. E. (2018). A meta-analysis of multicultural competencies and psychotherapy process and outcome. *Journal of Counseling Psychology*, *62*(3), 337–350. https://doi.org/10.1037/cou0000086

Torres, L., & Taknint, J. T. (2015). Ethnic microaggressions, traumatic stress symptoms, and latino depression: A moderated mediational model. *Journal of Counseling Psychology*, *62*, 393–401.

Vieten, C., Scammell, S., Pilato, R., Ammondson, I., Pargament, K. I., & Lukoff, D. (2013). Spiritual and religious competencies for psychologists. *Psychology of Religion and Spirituality*, *5*(3), 129–144. https://doi.org/10.1037/a0032699

Wampold, B. E., & Imel, Z. E. (2015). *The great psychotherapy debate* (2nd ed.). London: Routledge/Taylor & Francis Group.

Watkins, C. E., Jr, Hook, J. N., Owen, J., DeBlaere, C., Davis, D. E., & Van Tongeren, D. R. (2019). Multicultural orientation in psychotherapy supervision: Cultural humility, cultural comfort, and cultural opportunities. *American Journal of Psychotherapy*, *72*(2), 38–46.

Yeo, E., & Torres-Harding, S. R. (2021). Rupture resolution strategies and the impact of rupture on the working alliance after racial microaggressions in therapy. *Psychotherapy*, *58*(4), 460–471. https://doi.org/10.1037/pst0000372

Part 3

Innovations for 21st Century Psychotherapy: Practice, Supervision & Training

Chapter 10

Information Technology and Behavioural Healthcare in the 21st Century

Jeb Brown, Ashley Simon and Justin Turner

Abstract

The use of data in the twenty-first century to improve expert decision-making has radically transformed what it means to be an expert in multiple fields, including behavioural healthcare. This chapter summarises the impact on information technology on the field, including use of digital platforms to enable video therapy and online cognitive behavioural therapy programmes. The chapter is intended for practitioners seeking information on how to be a twenty-first century expert, where years of education and experience matter less compared to evidence of performance in the form of solid outcome data. Key to the use of outcome data is expertise in how to use questionnaires in therapy and how to interpret results, both at the individual client level as well as overall results across multiple clients. A twenty-first century expert measures are not simply to measure outcomes but to improve results over time. Failure to incorporate the use of data into routine practice ignores an evidence based practice with decades of evidence as to its effectiveness, potentially resulting in suboptimal care.

Keywords: Data-informed psychotherapy; technology; psychotherapy outcomes; online therapy; routine outcome monitoring; 21st centruy practitioners

Chapter Learning Outcomes

(1) Understand the history of information technology and advances in the management of outcomes in behavioural health services.
(2) Understand the implications for practitioners seeking to demonstrate expertise in the twenty-first century.

Evidence Based Counselling & Psychotherapy for the 21st Century Practitioner, 117–133

Published under exclusive licence by Emerald Publishing Limited
doi:10.1108/978-1-80455-732-720231010

Introduction

In this chapter, we will review and discuss the changes in the provision of psychotherapy and other behavioural health services that are occurring during the first quarter of the twenty-first century. The changes discussed have resulted from both advances in information technology in the field and society at large. This includes the use of data and decision support algorithms to inform clinical judgement, identify high value practitioners, and the use of digital platforms to deliver services. This chapter will spotlight these impacts upon the delivery of behavioural health services specifically.

Within the healthcare system of the United States, famous for its high cost and mediocre quality compared to healthcare systems in other developed countries (Kurani & Wager, 2021), much of the care is delivered by for-profit entities and funded by other for-profit entities providing health insurance. We will refer to these entities broadly as health plans. The result is that practitioners and health plans often argue about what constitutes appropriate care (medical necessity). Of course, money is easier to measure than outcome, so decisions are frequently driven by financial concerns, leaving the client caught in the middle. Despite the obvious downsides of this arrangement, the continued tension creates a fertile environment for innovation, research, and use of data to aid decision-making on all sides.

One of the authors (Brown) has been a part-time practicing psychologist until his recent retirement. Over his career, he spent 20 years in clinical management for increasingly large systems of care. In this capacity, he headed the development of the so-called clinical information systems to assist in the measurement of outcomes and manage costs across large networks of practitioners. The ultimate goal of a clinical information system is outcomes management along with cost management, thus increasing the value of services (Brown, 1994; Brown, Fraser, & Bendoraitis, 1995). A clinical information system differs from simple outcomes measurement programmes in that it has the capacity to incorporate diverse data sets from multiple sources while making it easy to query and generate output that is useful for decision support.

In 1997, Brown founded the Center for Clinical Informatics to provide consulting services for other large health plans and practitioners seeking to increase their use of data in the pursuit of value. In 2007, Brown and his long-time research colleague Takuya Minami, PhD, founded the ACORN collaboration, a clinical information system informed by a network of behavioural health clinics and funders of behavioural health services working together to measure and improve outcomes (Brown & Minami, 2009). At the time of this writing, the ACORN system contains 4.3 million completed outcome questionnaires, comprising 1.2 million episodes of care.

The system also contains cost data for hundreds of thousands of individuals receiving care paid for by health plans, as well as the credentialling information (training, years of experience, and licensure type) for tens of thousands behavioural health practitioners.

Turn of the Century Zeitgeist

The last few decades of the twentieth century were an exciting time for the behavioural health field. Here, in the United States, demand for services and funding were expanding, as were the number and types of licensed providers. New discoveries in both psychotherapy methods (evidence based treatments) as well as pharmacological treatments promised to radically transform the provision of care. Development of screening questionnaires to aid in the diagnosis and application of the most appropriate clinically proven treatment (psychotherapy and/or mediation) would lead to the improvement of outcomes for consumers of behavioural health services.

For most of the twentieth century, practitioners tended to belong to 'schools' of therapy. The schools were generally founded by creative and innovative practitioners/researchers who wrote persuasively and accumulated trainees and followers. These trainees and followers then often split with their mentor to pursue new directions and found new schools of therapy. The names are familiar, starting with Freud and his descendants. Practitioners in this era tended to associate their perceived personal effectiveness as being due in large part to their preferred school of therapy, the impact of supervision, ongoing training in the preferred treatment methods, and the expected effects of expertise gained over time.

But storm clouds were gathering over many of the prevailing assumptions about what constituted quality of care. Rapidly increasing use of digital technology in the field made possible the aggregation of data from multiple sources, ready for analyses by increasing powerful computers. It suddenly became possible to examine drivers of both cost and outcomes in the real world, and to pursue the optimisation of value, as defined by the outcome of care divided by the cost of care. How much improvement does every unit of cost buy, and how do we buy the most improvement at the best price?

At the end of the twentieth century, cost for behavioural healthcare in the United States was rising rapidly. Most insurance was obtained through one's place of employment. It should be no surprise that employers began to ask 'Need we spend so much money?' For-profit providers of insurance offered to supply a solution, and thus was born 'managed care coverage', where services were provided within a defined network of providers, and many procedures and treatments required prior approval. This proved particularly attractive for behavioural healthcare, where sessions could be approved and reapproved at frequent intervals based on clinical criteria for medical necessity.

Revolution in Models of Understanding

At the turn of the century, American/Israeli psychologist Daniel Kahneman (2002 Nobel Prize in Economics), his colleague Amos Tversky, as well as others, began to investigate cognitive basis for common human errors that arise from heuristics and biases (Kahneman, 2011). What it meant to be an expert in most fields began to experience a radical shift around this time, from sports to investing to medicine. For just about any major field where money was involved, it was no longer enough for experts to just have a wealth of personal experience in their field. Experts were now falling behind their peers if they weren't also making use of data and predictive modelling to augment decision-making and reduce the effect of individual heuristics and biases.

The beginning of aggregate data in behavioural health began with Smith and Glass (1977), who published what was the first of many meta-analyses of treatment outcomes for psychotherapy. They combined the results of 375 controlled evaluations of psychotherapy to estimate the overall effectiveness of the practice. The methodology was innovative and established one of the first benchmarks for the effectiveness of psychotherapy as a whole.

Smith and Glass utilised a statistic commonly known as effect size. The use of this statistic, known technically as Cohen's *d* (Cohen, 1988) is now standard when reporting results of individual studies as well as meta-analyses. For purposes of this chapter, the use of effect size can be thought of as the difference between the intake score on the outcome measure and the last score obtained in treatment (pre–post change) divided by the standard deviation of the outcome measure at intake. Different populations have different intake scores and standard deviations. Effect size works best for purposes of comparison to those subjects or clients with intake scores in a so-called 'clinical range', which tends to be calculated somewhere close to the those in upper 25% of severity of symptom scores when sampling a general population of individuals who have never been in therapy. For those seeking therapy, about 75% fall into the clinical range.

Calculation of effect size is also subject to regression artefacts (Campbell & Kenny, 2002). Subjects with scores further from the mean exhibit more change than those close to the mean. When comparing smaller samples, or very different populations, this makes the use of simple effect size problematic. For this reason, effect size scores reported from the ACORN sample have been adjusted for severity and is referred to as a severity adjusted effect size (SAES; Lambert, Minami, Hamilton, McCulloch, et al., 2009).

An effect size of 1 means the individual improved one standard deviation on the questionnaire. When rounded to the nearest tenth, the average effect size for outpatient psychotherapy (often combined with medications) is 0.8. This would seem like a bold generalisation, but it is a fact backed up by four decades of research since the Smith and Glass article, where the effect size was estimated to be right around 0.8, depending on the type of comparison. Remarkably, there is no evidence that effect sizes are increasing across virtually all methods of therapy with an adequate research base to be included in the meta-analyses. All appear to produce equivalent results. (Wampold & Imel, 2015). Keep in mind that 0.8 is a robust effect size and can be considered evidence of highly effective treatment (McCloud, 2019).

Another interesting finding using effect size comes from the psychopharmacology world. Meta-analysis of drug company-sponsored trials of antidepressants showed large effect sizes for the placebo condition. Kirsch et al. (2008) obtained data for all studies on antidepressants conducted by pharmaceutical companies for the Food and Drug Administration, regardless of whether they were published. In total, only 52% of the studies showed a statistically significant difference in favour of the active drug. These studies were virtually all published, while very few of those that failed to show superiority of the drug made it into peer reviewed journals. When Kirsch and colleagues provided a new meta-analysis including all available data, the advantage of medication all but disappeared, and could hardly be judged as clinically meaningful (Kirsch, 2009).

If psychotherapy is not becoming more effective, all well-researched methods of therapy seem to have equivalent results, and some of the most commonly prescribed drugs appear not to work much better than placebo, then what is going on? Based on this, how can we improve outcomes? Clearly, it's time for a paradigm shift, a new way to understand what the clients are communicating through the data they give us.

Clinical Information Systems

Ideally, a clinical information system provides a coherent and consistent structure to extract information from multiple sources of raw data while at the same time permitting a degree of random creativity and experimentation. The information extracted from the data is used to develop clinical algorithms which serve as decision support tools (Brown et al., 1995). A state-of-the-art clinical information system needs to meet the following criteria:

- Flexibility in the choice of questionnaires.
- Capacity to handle very large data sets containing tens of millions records.
- Ready integration of useful data from multiple external sources.
    - Cost data
        - Mental health services and costs
        - Medical services and costs
        - Pharmacy data on drugs, dosage, refill history, and prescriber.
    - Practitioner credentialling data
- Ready availability of state-of-the-art analytic software to query data and analyse data.
- Flexible creation of reports and graphs.
- Continuous data mining to develop decision support tools based on a number on variables.
- Provide end users including practitioner's easy access to decision support information useful to perform their jobs effectively, as measured by results.

One of the authors (Brown) was employed for five years in the mid-1990s as the Director of Clinical Operations for AETNA US Healthcare, with an estimated 23 million lives covered at that time (Eaton, 1996). He was responsible for overseeing the literature reviews and the creation of diagnostic specific treatment guidelines to be disseminated to providers, supposedly providing evidence of 'what works' (Brown, 1994; Brown, Dreis, & Nace, 1999).

Pressure from employers to cut costs was an ever-present demand. Corporate funding was available to assemble a team of researchers, statisticians, and IT professionals to develop what was perhaps the first clinical information system dedicated to behavioural healthcare (Brown et al., 1995; Brown & Kornmayer, 1996; Lambert & Brown, 1996). Outside academic consultants who became members of the team included Michael Lambert, PhD, and Gary Burlingame, PhD, both psychotherapy researchers at Brigham Young University. In 1997, Brown formed an independent consulting firm to assist in the development of clinical information systems for other health plans. Fortunately, he was able to enlist the collaboration and to add new members to the team, including Bruce Wampold, PhD from the University of Wisconsin and one of his doctoral students in the counselling psychology graduate programme, Takuya Minami.

One of their first projects was for PacifiCare Health Systems, which was later acquired by United Health Care, which continued the work on the clinical information system, then known as the ALERT system. Michael Lambert at that time was well known for his work on the so-called common factors in psychotherapy (Lambert, 1993). Bruce Wampold's (2001) first book, *The Great Psychotherapy Debate* (first edition), was threatening to shake the foundations of how those in the behavioural healthcare profession thought about psychotherapy and what really made a difference in outcome. Based on a review of over 40 years of psychotherapy research, Wampold concluded that the method of psychotherapy made very little difference in outcomes and that the largest source of variance was the individual practitioner.

The use of these comprehensive clinical information systems made it possible to improve outcomes by providing practitioners with decision support while using practitioner profiling to increase referrals to effective practitioners. This had the effect of not only improving outcomes, but also decreasing costs, thereby dramatically increasing the value of the services.

The following section describes in greater detail the history of twenty-first century evolving methodology for creating questionnaires, investigating predictors of outcome, and appropriate models for practitioner profiling with regard to outcome, cost, and value.

Where's the Variance?

By this time, the research team had access to data from a variety of questionnaires, some of which were created by members of the team (Burlingame, Jasper, et al., 2001; Burlingame, Mosier, et al., 2001; Lambert, Gregersen, & Burlingame, 2004; Lambert, Hatfield, et al., 2001). The team also searched the literature for results of analyses of other questionnaires, and in particular, the search for underlying factors. Questionnaires are often judged and selected based on face validity as a measure of depression, anxiety, quality of social relationships, functionality in day-to-day activities, etc. However, from a psychometric point of view, a better estimate of validity is construct validity, as determined using factor analysis.

Factor analysis revealed that the items with face validity for depression, anxiety, social relationships, and day-to-day functioning all loaded on a common factor. They also all tended to improve at the same rate. This meant that questionnaires could be shortened to an extent without sacrificing construct validity, reliability, or sensitivity to change. For example, it is possible to create a 15 item questionnaire with a reliability (Chronbach's coefficient alpha) of 0.9, while a 30 item questionnaire with similar item content might have a reliability of 0.93 and a 45 item questionnaire a reliability of 0.94. That said, reliability of a questionnaire begins to degrade significantly if you take this to the extreme. A questionnaire with less than 5 items is likely to have a reliability of under 0.73, for example.

What About the Individual Practitioner?

Perhaps the most important article to come out of this collaboration was Wampold and Brown (2005), which employed what was at that time an underused statistical method known as hierarchical linear modelling. This permitted the research team to identify how much of the variance in outcomes was due to the individual practitioner, exploring practitioner variables such as advanced degree type, years of experience, as well as controlling for client variables such as severity of symptoms at intake, diagnosis, age, sex, and length of treatment.

The largest source of variance in the treatment outcomes was the individual practitioner, and yet practitioner subvariables such as graduate degree and years of experience were unrelated to outcome. The distribution of effect sizes for practitioners was normally distributed, with large and clinically meaningful differences between practitioners with above average results compared to those with below average outcomes.

What About the Medications?

Also, this study looked at the effects for antidepressant medications by practitioners' outcomes for clients receiving psychotherapy alone versus those receiving psychotherapy plus medication. Outcomes were evaluated at the practitioner level, so that it was possible to compare each practitioner's results with or without medication. It should come as no surprise at this point to learn that the individual practitioner was the single largest predictor of outcomes. For those clients seen by practitioners with below average therapy results, the addition of a medication did not improve results at all. While practitioners with above average therapy results had clients who also showed strong improvement on medications, the difference between psychotherapy alone versus those receiving psychotherapy plus medication was not clinically meaningful.

Wampold and his colleagues quickly published a study confirming this finding (Kim, Wampold, & Bolt, 2006; McKay, Imel, & Wampold, 2006). They reanalysed data from the well-known National Institute of Mental Health funded study of treatments for depression and in particular, data from the medication only placebo control leg of the study. The nine different psychiatrists who treated the clients were blinded to whether they received the active medication or placebo. The authors found that 9% of the variance of outcome was due to the psychiatrist and only 3% to the medication. The top third of psychiatrists had a better outcome with placebo than the bottom third had with the active medication.

This suggests that there was something about the person of the psychiatrist that mediated placebo response, just as there was something about the therapist that mediated the response to both psychotherapy and medication.

The finding that the largest source of variance in outcomes is the individual clinician leads to the obvious conclusion that one of the fastest ways to improve outcomes across a large network of psychotherapy providers was to find ways to increase referrals to providers with good outcomes. The methodology for benchmarking practitioners' outcomes will be discussed in a following section, but first it's useful to look at the effects for measurement and feedback.

Measurement and Feedback to Improve Outcomes

Other researchers were already experimenting with predicting expected change to identify clients failing to improve early in treatment. They found early failure to improve was associated with a poor outcome (Wolfgang, Lowry, Kopta, Einstein, & Howard, 2001; Wolfgang, Martinovich, & Howard, 1999). Following their lead, the team developed predictive models to identify which clients were at risk, the so-called 'off track' clients. Algorithms were quickly developed to both provide feedback to clinicians and to care managers. Rather than asking care managers to review every case, their efforts were focussed on the roughly 15% of cases that were deemed at risk. Continuing care was authorised automatically for the others.

Is Client Data a Better Predictor of Outcome than the Clinician's judgement?

The team initially asks practitioners to also rate client symptoms. If the client reported improvement, the provider rating tended to agree. However, if the client completed questionnaire indicated a significant increase in symptoms, the provider ratings still indicated improvement, just not as much. Another finding was the provider's description of their method of therapy had no relationship with the outcome or length of therapy. This was very much in keeping with findings by reported by Lambert et al. (2002) and Wampold (2001).

Michael Lambert began to test the effects of measurement and feedback in the counselling centre and Brigham Young University (BYU). The series of studies from his team at BYU confirmed that outcomes were significantly improved for 'off track' cases in the condition where clinician received this feedback from the questionnaires as opposed to the no feedback condition (Lambert, Hunt, & Vermeersch, 2003; Lambert, Whipple, et al., 2001; Lambert et al., 2002).

The process of routine measurement and feedback (discussed briefly in a previous chapter) has been referred to by various names such as feedback-informed treatment (FIT), routine outcomes measurement (ROM), and outcomes-informed care (OIC). This rapidly expanding area of research quickly spawned a number of commercial products designed to facilitate routine outcomes measurement and feedback. These outcomes management systems differ from a true clinical information system as they are constructed to utilise a discrete set of copyrighted questionnaires and lack the capacity to rapidly integrate multiple sources or to use multivariate statistics to predict expected change (Barkham, Mellor-Clark, &

Stiles, 2015; Boswell, Kraus, Castonguay, & Youn, 2015; Duncan, 2015; Kopta, 2015; Lambert, 2015).

Measurement 2.0 and the ACORN Collaboration

In 2007, Brown and Minami headed the development of a new clinical information system intended to be shared by any interested collaborating organisations and funded by health plans and clinics utilising the system. This became known as the ACORN Toolkit (Brown, Simon, Cameron, & Minami, 2015). Warren Lambert, PhD, an expert psychometrician teaching at Vanderbilt University joined the collaboration and headed the effort to develop and document methodologies for questionnaires development, calculation of SAES, and the benchmarking of practitioners' individual outcomes. The methodology was documented in a white paper coauthored by researchers and health plan administrators associated with the project and was entitled Outcomes Measurement 2.0 (Lambert et al., 2009).

The ACORN platform was designed to enable the use of any questionnaire made with validated items (correlation with the common factor at 0.5 or higher). A methodology for rapid development and validation of questionnaires was needed. This became known as the 'item torture test' (the idea being that each available item is submitted to a variety of psychometric tests based on both classical test theory and item response theory).

These included:

- distribution of item response scores at intake;
- item loading on specific factors of interest;
- the slope of change over time in therapy; and
- ability to items or particular interest for risk management.

The team also evaluated different item response formats, such as Likert response scales using three, four, five or more options as well as visual analogue scales, which asks clients to mark a response on a continuous line. The team concluded that the traditional five-point Likert scale produced excellent results. Another innovation was to abbreviate the items by using a common preface such as 'How often in the past two weeks did you …' and only partial sentences for the item itself (i.e. 'did you feel sad'). This resulted in questionnaires that were much quicker to administer. With this information on each item, specific questionnaires with predicable psychometric qualities can be created as needed, since the properties of the scales on a questionnaire are essentially a combination of the properties of the individual items on a scale. Development of reliable and valid questionnaires designed to target specific populations and to meet the needs of clinicians using the system followed.

At the same time a separate group of psychometric researchers were developing questionnaires for use in the DSM-IV to measure outcomes for various populations and diagnoses. They used the same methodology, including five-point Likert scales and use of partial sentences for items (American Psychiatric Association, DSMV-TR-Online Assessment Measures). This methodology is also consistent with the American Psychological Association guidelines on the use of questionnaires, which states in Guideline 6:

> Psychologists who conduct psychological testing, assessment, and evaluation endeavor to select
>
> (a) assessment tools that demonstrate sufficient validity evidence for their uses, sufficient score reliability, and sound psychometric properties
> (b) measures that are fair and appropriate for the evaluation purpose, population, setting, and context at hand.

Questionnaires were designed to have a reliability of approximately 0.8 with sensitivity to change over time. This resulted in questionnaires that were significantly shorter to use with some outcomes measurement exhibiting similar excellent psychometric properties. Some outcomes measurement systems encouraged the use of very short questionnaires with as few as four items to increase clinician acceptance. However, ultra-brief questionnaires sacrifice both reliability and the ability to sample specific symptoms of interest. The ACORN experience suggests strongly that questionnaires that could be completed in less than two minutes are acceptable to practitioners and clients, without the need to be ultra-short.

The collaboration also developed and tested brief scales to allow the client to provide feedback on the so-called therapeutic alliance. As conceptualised by Wampold and Imel (2015), alliance consisted of three elements: agreement on the nature of the problem, agreement of the approach to solving the problem, and client's perception of warmth, empathy, and acceptance by the clinician. ACORN questionnaires typically included at least three alliance items. Initially, clinicians were encouraged to ask clients to complete an outcome questionnaire at the start of the session and an alliance questionnaire at the end of the session to receive feedback on the session. Quite early in the collaboration, it became evident that if the client completed an alliance measure, the outcomes were significantly better.

The outcome questionnaires were often administered by front office staff and then made available to the clinician after completion by the client. This resulted in a high consistency of administration of the outcome questionnaires while it also became apparent that many clinicians neglected to ask the client to complete an alliance questionnaire. Based on feedback from various participants in the collaboration, ACORN began to include the alliance items on the questionnaires administered at the start of the session asking the client to look back at the prior session. This provided the clinicians with alliance feedback at the start of session while also greatly increasing completion of the alliance scale, resulting in a significant improvement in outcomes. In a short period of time, almost all the participating clinics within the ACORN collaboration adapted the use of outcome questionnaires with the alliance items included. The ACORN collaboration also built on the benchmarking methodology published by members of the collaboration, and in particular Takuya Minami (Minami, Serlin, Wampold, Kircher, & Brown, 2008; Minami, Wampold, et al., 2008; Minami, Wampold, Serlin, Kircher, & Brown, 2007). These provided the basis for the methodology employed within ACORN for evaluating and displaying the practitioner's overall results.

ACORN-generated Research

Initially, research findings within the ACORN collaboration were distributed within the collaboration without submission to peer reviewed journals. Results and instructional videos based on ACORN research were distributed via the ACORN collaboration website and login page for the Toolkit. More recently, results have been published in a series of articles published in the online journal of *Society for the Advancement of Psychotherapy*. This journal is geared towards practicing therapists rather than an academic audience and has proven to be a useful means to distribute findings to members of the collaboration. A number of these online articles are referenced for readers wishing to dig deeper into findings reported in this chapter.

Brown, Simon, and Minami (2015) in a provocatively titled article (Are you any good as a therapist?) published the distribution of clinicians' SAESs as well as demonstrating how to adjust for sample size. Part of the ACORN strategy to improve clinician results has been to provide direct feedback on their overall effectiveness. This appears to be particularly important in encouraging and aiding clinicians in improving individual results.

When attempting to compare results between individual clinicians, it is necessary to use multivariate statistics to account for differences in diagnoses, age, sex, and severity of symptoms at intake, as measured by the intake score on the outcome questionnaire. Of these variables, the intake score is by far the strongest predictor of change in therapy, followed by diagnosis which accounts for a small but still significant percentage of variance. For this reason, the ACORN collaboration pioneered the use of what is referred to as a SAES, which provides an effect size estimated after controlling for case mix variables (Brown, Simon, Cameron, & Minami, 2015; Lambert et al., 2009).

It became apparent that the frequency with which clinicians viewed their data was strongly associated with how much they improved their results from one year to the next (Brown, Cazauvieilh, & Simon, 2021; Brown, Simon, & Foster, 2021). If clinician login counts per month reached a certain threshold, clinician results tended to improve. If not, the clinicians tended to show no improvement from one year to the next. Of course, the degree of improvement was also dependent of the clinician's effect size in the prior year. During a baseline period of two years, clinicians in the bottom quartile for outcomes exhibited an average gain in their effect size of 0.17 (from 0.60 to 0.77). Clinicians in the middle two quartiles averaged a 0.12 gain in their already strong effect sizes (from 0.85 to 0.97). For those in the upper quartile in the baseline period, with an already exceptionally large average effect size of 1.16, results tended to stay stable in the subsequent year regardless of log in frequency.

Within the ACORN collaboration, clinical supervisors and agency leadership can monitor practitioners' mean SAES and how often they log in. This clinical oversight encourages more active engagement by the clinicians with viewing and understanding their data. The admin staff and clinical supervisors are critical to encouraging practitioners to use measurement and feedback to improve personal results.

The routine collection of alliance data along with the outcome data allowed research collaborators to explore the relationship between alliance and outcome. The results point to the complexity of understanding how to best use alliance measures. Having a near perfect alliance score at every session is NOT associated with the best outcomes. Rather, clients who rate the alliance as less than perfect early in treatment are likely to report significantly more symptom improvement if alliance scores improve over the course the treatment. Apparently, the critical skill for the clinician is to encourage the client to provide accurate and useful feedback, not simply allow the client to reassure the clinician that all is well. This finding is particularly true for treatment that is relatively short term (Mahon, Brown, & Simon, 2021a, 2021b).

Emerging Technologies for Delivering Behavioural Healthcare

The use of the so-called telemedicine was expanding during the twenty-first century, particularly useful for expanding services to more remote communities. However, the overall impact on psychotherapy services was minimal until the COVID-19 pandemic, which resulted in rapid transition in societal behaviour to minimise human contact and limit the risk of the transmission. ACORN accommodated this shift to teletherapy via enhancing options for administering questionnaires via online links which could be emailed or texted to clients prior to sessions. The various questionnaires in use were modified to include an item indicating to whether the session was in-person or via video. Since March 2020 to the time of this writing (June 2022), the ACORN database accumulated outcome data for 52,504 clients entering treatment with intake scores in a clinical range of distress. Their mean effect size was 0.86, well into the highly effective range.

This rich data set permitted the research team to dig deeper, exploring the relative effectiveness of purely face-to-face therapy compared to purely video therapy, as well as a combination of the two. The data also permitted an exploration in differences between youth and adults in their response to video therapy. The results were illuminating. For adults, a combination of in-person and video therapy resulted in a more sessions and a larger SAES than either in-person or video therapy alone ($p<0.01$). For youth, the results were even more striking. Video therapy alone or in combination with in-person therapy resulted in significantly longer engagement in treatment and larger SAES than in-person only ($p<0.01$). There was an average of over 0.3 greater effect sizes for those receiving teletherapy in combination with in-person therapy (Simon, Brown, & Turner, 2021). This is clearly a robust result and suggests that video therapy has an important role to play in the delivery of services.

The first two decades of the twenty-first century also saw introduction of websites offering some form of an internet-based cognitive behavioural therapy self-guided approach to therapy. Ed Jones, PhD, a long-time collaborator and contributor to ACORN in his roles as a senior executive in different health plans is currently a consultant to Learn to Live, a company that offers iCBT lessons targeted towards depression and anxiety. Dr Jones led the efforts to utilise this rich source of outcome data on iCBT to look for clues on how to improve results. Learn to Live asks users to complete an outcome questionnaire at the start of each online lesson, permitting an estimate of effect size and comparison of outcomes to those of outpatient psychotherapy as benchmarked using the ACORN data. The goal was to achieve results comparable to in-person therapy. At first, it was not clear how this was possible.

Initial analyses of the data indicated that improvement was superior to outpatient therapy if the user completed all seven lessons of the programme. However, only 16% of users completed all the lessons. About 56% completed the programme in three or fewer sessions. Also, the session-to-session change was greater in earlier sessions of outpatient therapy, resulting in an overall effect size for Learn to Live users of 0.46 compared to 0.74 for the outpatient therapy sample (Brown, Jones, & Cazauvieilh, 2020). Learn to Live also includes the option for users to receive additional support in the form of the so-called coaching by Learn to Live staff counsellors, automated texts with 'mindfulness', and enlisting friends or family members as the so-called 'teammates' to provide additional support and encouragement. Analyses revealed that increasing provided social support was a pathway to improved results. This provided the basis for a quality improvement (QI) initiative to encourage the use of the coaching and other support options, resulting in a significant increase in the use of one of the support options (from 49% to 65%) and an accompanying increase in mean effect size. All users receiving the additional support reported results equal to or greater than those of the ACORN benchmarks for outpatient therapy. The combined conditions of personal coaching and mindfulness texts had the largest effect size of 1.1 compared to 0.74 for the ACORN sample. The increased use of the supports resulted in an overall company effect size of 0.83 prior to the follow-up evaluation of the QI initiative (Brown & Jones, 2022a).

The large sample available after the follow-up period also permitted the evaluation of the least utilised form of additional support, the so-called 'teammates' option, asking the user to list additional sources of support such as friends, family members, or coworkers. While only 8% of the users had selected this option, the results were dramatic with an effect size >0.8. If combined with the coaching options, the effect size increases to 1.1. Interestingly, the results were not due to completing more lessons. Rather, users reported significantly greater improvement between lessons (Brown & Jones, 2022b).

Conclusion

At this point in the twenty-first century, research on what constitutes expertise in the provision of psychotherapy services involves the use of routine outcomes measure, feedback, and other decision support tools. Practitioner assessments of their own expertise in the absence of data is not sufficient, can result in over-confidence, and provides no means to gauge improvement. In fact, one study found that 0% of practitioners judged their results to be below average (Walfish, McAlister, O'Donnell, & Lambert, 2012). Failure to measure outcomes can be viewed as suboptimal care. Tracey, Wampold, Goodyear, and Lichtenberg (2015) redefined clinical expertise to include the practitioner's routine use of measurement in an ongoing effort to improve results. Furthermore, practitioners without evidence of their own effectiveness will find it increasingly difficult to compete in a world increasingly using data to establish the value of services.

The widespread adaptation of alternative delivery systems offers promise but lacks consistency in results. The similar proliferation of companies offering video therapy offers the promise of increased access to affordable services. However, many such companies are actively recruiting providers without the screening and interview that might occur if they were applying for a job at a clinic or to become part of the healthcare network. One lesson seems clear: the active use of outcomes measurement and other data for quality improvement, along with an increased level of transparency with regard to results, is critical to continued progress in our field and the assurance of the best care possible to consumers of behavioural health services.

References

ACORN Collaboration Website. Retrieved from https://acorncollaboration.org/

American Psychiatric Association, DSMV-TR-Online Assessment Measures. Retrieved from https://www.psychiatry.org/psychiatrists/practice/dsm/educational-resources/assessment-measures#section_17

Barkham, M., Mellor-Clark, J., & Stiles, W. B. (2015). A CORE approach to progress monitoring and feedback: Enhancing evidence and improving practice. *Psychotherapy*, *52*(4), 402–411.

Boswell, J. F., Kraus, D. R., Castonguay, L. G., & Youn, S. J. (2015). Treatment outcome package: Measuring and facilitating multidimensional change. *Psychotherapy*, *52*(4), 422–431.

Brown, G. S. (1994). What are "good" guidelines? *Behavioral Health Management*, *14*(5), 6–9.

Brown, G. S., Cazauvieilh, C., & Simon, A. (2021). Clinician engagement in feedback informed care and patient outcomes [Web article]. Retrieved from http://www.societyforpsychotherapy.org/clinician-engagement-in-feedback-informed-care-and-patient-outcomes

Brown, G. S., Dreis, S., & Nace, D. (1999). What really makes a difference in psychotherapy outcomes? And why does managed care want to know? In S. Miller & M. Hubble (Eds.), *Heart and soul of change* (pp. 389–406). Washington, DC: American Psychological Association Press.

Brown, G. S., Fraser, J. B., & Bendoraitis, T. M. (1995). Transforming the future – The coming impact of clinical information systems. *Behavioral Health Management*, *14*(5), 8–12.

Brown, G. S., & Jones, E. (2022a). Improving results for digital therapeutics [Web article]. Retrieved from http://www.societyforpsychotherapy.org/improving-results-for-digital-therapeutics

Brown, G. S., & Jones, E. (2022b). Improving results for digital therapeutics with social support [Web article]. Retrieved from http://www.societyforpsychotherapy.org/improving-results-for-digital-therapeutics-with-social-support

Brown, G. S., Jones, E., & Cazauvieilh, C. (2020, May). Effectiveness for online cognitive behavioral therapy versus outpatient treatment: A session by session analysis [Web article]. Retrieved from http://www.societyforpsychotherapy.org/effectiveness-for-online-cognitive-behavioral-therapy-versus-outpatient-treatment

Brown, G. S., & Kornmayer, K. (1996). Expert systems restructure managed care practice: Implementation and practice. *Behavioral Health Care Tomorrow*, *5*(1), 31–34.

Brown, G. S., & Minami, T. (2009). Outcomes management, reimbursement, and the future of psychotherapy. In S. Miller & M. Hubble (Eds.), *Heart and soul of change*. Washington, DC: American Psychological Association Press.

Brown, G. S., Simon, A. E., Cameron, J., & Minami, T. (2015). A collaborative outcome resource network (ACORN): Tools for increasing the value of psychotherapy. *Psychotherapy*, *52*(4), 412–421. https://doi.org/10.1037/pst0000033

Brown, G. S., Simon, A., & Foster, L. (2021). Clinical impact of school-based interventions [Web article]. Retrieved from http://www.societyforpsychotherapy.org/clinical-impact-of-school-based-interventions

Brown, G. S., Simon, A. E., & Minami, T. (2015). Are you any good … as a therapist? [Web article]. Retrieved from http://www.societyforpsychotherapy.org/are-you-any-good-as-a-therapist

Burlingame, G. M., Jasper, B. W., Peterson, G., Wells, M. G., Lambert, M. J., Reisinger, C. W., & Brown, G. S. (2001). *Administration and scoring manual for the YLSQ*. Wilmington, DC: American Professional Credentialing Services.

Burlingame, G. M., Mosier, J., Wells, M., Atkin, Q., Lambert, M., Whoolery, M., & Latkowski, M. (2001). Tracking the influence of mental health treatment: The development of the youth outcome questionnaire. *Clinical Psychology & Psychotherapy*, *8*, 361–379. doi:10.1002/cpp.315

Campbell, D. T., & Kenny, D. A. (2002). *A primer on regression artifacts*. New York, NY: Guildford. ISBN 9781572308596.

Cohen, J. (1988). *Statistical power analysis for the behavioral sciences* (2nd ed.). Hillsdale, NJ: Erlbaum.

Duncan, B. (2015). The partners for change outcome management system (PCOMS) revisiting the client's frame of reference. *Psychotherapy*, *52*(4), 391–401.

Eaton, L. K. (1996). Aetna to buy U.S. Healthcare in a big move to managed care. *New York Times*. Retrieved from https://www.nytimes.com/1996/04/02/business/aetna-to-buy-us-healthcare-in-big-move-to-managed-care.html

Kahneman, D. (2011). *Thinking, fast and slow*. New York, NY: Farrar, Straus and Giroux. ISBN 978-0374275631

Kim, D. M., Wampold, B. E., & Bolt, D. M. (2006). Therapist effects in psychotherapy: A random-effects modeling of the National Institute of Mental Health Treatment of Depression Collaborative Research Program data. *Psychotherapy Research, 16*(02), 161–172.

Kirsch, I. (2009). *The emperor's new drugs: Exploding the anti-depressant myth*. New York, NY: The Random House Group. ISBN 978-0465020164

Kirsch, I., Deacon, B. J., Huedo-Medina, T. B., Scoboria, A., Moore, T. J., & Johnson, B. T. (2008). Initial severity and antidepressant benefits: A meta-analysis of data submitted to the food and drug administration. *PLoS Medicine*, *5*, 260–268.

Kopta, M. (2015). Measuring psychotherapy outcomes with the behavioral health measure–20: Efficient and comprehensive. *Psychotherapy*, *52*(4), 442–448.

Kurani, N., & Wager, E. (2021). How does the quality of the U.S. health system compare to other countries? Retrieved from https://www.healthsystemtracker.org/chart-collection/quality-u-s-healthcare-system-compare-countries/

Lambert, M. J. (1993). Common factors in psychotherapy. In A. Bergin & S. Garfield (Eds.), *Handbook of psychotherapy and behavior change*. New York, NY: John Wiley and Sons, Inc. ISBN 978-0471545132

Lambert, M. J. (2015). Progress feedback and the OQ-system: The past and the future. *Psychotherapy*, *52*(4), 381–390.

Lambert, M. J., & Brown, G. S. (1996). Data-based management for tracking outcome in private practice. *Clinical Psychology: Science and Practice*, *14*(2), 172–178.

Lambert, M. J., Gregersen, A. T., & Burlingame, G. M. (2004). The outcome questionnaire-45. In M. E. Maruish (Ed.), *The use of psychological testing for treatment planning and outcomes assessment: Instruments for adults* (pp. 191–234). London: Lawrence Erlbaum Associates Publishers.

Lambert, M. J., Hatfield, D. R., Vermeersch, D. A., Burlingame, G. M., Reisinger, C. W., & Brown, G. S. (2001). *Administration and scoring manual for the LSQ*. Wilmington, DC: American Professional Credentialing Services.

Lambert, M. J., Hunt, R. D., & Vermeersch, D. (2003). Optimizing outcome through prediction and measurement of psychological functioning. In *Core processes in brief psychodynamic psychotherapy: Advancing effective practice* (pp. 23–45).

Lambert, M. J., Whipple, J. L., Smart, D. W., Vermeersch, D., Nielsen, S., & Hawkins, E. (2001). The effects of providing therapists with feedback on patient progress during psychotherapy: Are outcomes enhanced? *Psychotherapy Research*, *11*, 49–68.

Lambert, M. J., Whipple, J., Vermeersch, D., Smart, D., Hawkins, E., Nielsen, S., & Goates, M. (2002). Enhancing psychotherapy outcomes via providing feedback on client progress: A replication. *Clinical Psychology & Psychotherapy*, *9*, 91–103. doi:10.1002/cpp.324

Lambert, W., Minami, T., Hamilton, E., McCulloch, J., Peters, J., Selway, M., Graves, C., Cameron, J., Brown, J. (2009). Outcomes measurement 2.0: Emerging technologies for managing treatment outcomes in behavioral healthcare. Retrieved from https://acorncollaboration.org/outcomes-20

Learn to Live Website. Retrieved from https://www.learntolive.com/

Lewis, M. (2016). *The undoing project: A friendship that changed our minds*. New York, NY: W. W. Norton & Company. ISBN 978-0606275644

Mahon, D., Brown, G. S., & Simon, A. (2021a). The relationship between session-to-session change on a therapeutic alliance measure and outcomes of treatment for short term psychotherapy [Web article]. Retrieved from https://societyforpsychotherapy.org/the-relationship-between-session-to-session-change-on-a-therapeutic-alliance-measure-and-outcome-of-treatment-for-short-term-psychotherapy/

Mahon, D., Brown, G. S., & Simon, A. (2021b). The relationship between measures of alliance and outcome in psychotherapy lasting more than five sessions [Web article]. Retrieved from https://societyforpsychotherapy.org/the-relationship-between-measures-of-alliance-and-outcome-in-psychotherapy-lasting-more-than-five-sessions/

McCloud, P. (2019). What does effect size tell you? Retrieved from https://www.simplypsychology.org/effect-size.html

McKay, K. M., Imel, Z. E., & Wampold, B. E. (2006). Psychiatrist effects in the psychopharmacological treatment of depression. *Journal of Affective Disorders*, *92*(2–3), 287–290.

Minami, T., Serlin, R. C., Wampold, B. E., Kircher, J. C., & Brown, G. S. (2008). Using clinical trials to benchmark effects produced in clinical practice. *Quality & Quantity*, *42*, 513–525.

Minami, T., Wampold, B. E., Serlin, R. C., Hamilton, E. G., Brown, G. S., & Kircher, J. C. (2008). Benchmarking the effectiveness of psychotherapy treatment for adult depression in a managed care environment. *Journal of Consulting and Clinical Psychology*, *76*, 116–124.

Minami, T., Wampold, B. E., Serlin, R. C., Kircher, J. C., & Brown, G. S. (2007). Benchmarks for psychotherapy efficacy in adult major depression. *Journal of Consulting and Clinical Psychology*, *75*, 232–243.

Simon, A. E., Brown, G. S., & Turner, J. K. (2021). Outcomes and alliance results of teletherapy versus in-person therapy [Web article]. Retrieved from https://acorn-collaboration.org/blog/2021/9/13/outcomes-and-alliance-results-of-teletherapy-versus-in-person-therapy

Smith, M. L., & Glass, G. V. (1977). Meta-analysis of psychotherapy outcome studies. *American Psychologist*, *32*(9), 752–760.

Tavakol, M., & Dennick, R. (2011). Making sense of Chronbach's alpha. *International Journal of Medical Education*, *2*, 53–55. Retrieved from https://www.ncbi.nlm.nih.gov/pmc/articles/PMC4205511/

Tracey, T. J. G., Wampold, B. E., Goodyear, R. K., & Lichtenberg, J. W. (2015). Improving expertise in psychotherapy. *Psychotherapy Bulletin*, *50*(1), 7–13.

Walfish, S., McAlister, B., O'Donnell, P., & Lambert, M. J. (2012). An investigation of self-assessment bias in mental health providers. *Psychological Reports*, *110*, 639–644. doi:10.2466/02.07.17.PR0.110.2.639-644

Wampold, B. E. (2001). *The great psychotherapy debate: Models, methods, and findings*. Hilsdale, NJ: Lawrence Erlbaum Associates Publishers.

Wampold, B. E., & Brown, G. S. (J.). (2005). Estimating variability in outcomes attributable to therapists: A naturalistic study of outcomes in managed care. J*ournal of Consulting and Clinical Psychology*, *73*(5), 914–923. https://doi.org/10.1037/0022-006X.73.5.914

Wampold, B., & Imel, Z. (2015). *The great psychotherapy debate: The evidence for what makes psychotherapy work*. New York, NY: Routledge. ISBN 978-0805857092 (First edition 2001).

Wolfgang, L., Lowry, J., Kopta, S., Einstein, D. & Howard, K. (2001). Prediction of dose–response relations based on patient characteristics. *Journal of Clinical Psychology*. *57*, 889–900.

Wolfgang, L., Martinovich, Z., & Howard, K. (1999). Patient profiling: An application of random coefficient regression models to depicting the response of a patient to outpatient psychotherapy. *Journal of Consulting and Clinical Psychology*, *67*, 571–577. doi:10.1037/0022-006X.67.4.571

Chapter 11

Deliberate Practice for Enhancing Skill Development in 21st Century Psychotherapy

Daryl Mahon

Abstract

Deliberate practice (DP) is an innovative training method for improving psychotherapy skills acquisition and expertise in the twenty-first century. I introduce the reader to the principles and processes of DP and the rationale for its use. The concept of DP is not new, indeed it is used to support the improvement of performance in diverse areas, from sport to music. However, its application to psychotherapy is still in its infancy. Firstly, I provide the rationale for including DP as a method of therapist training based on research that illustrates that many of the current criteria that we use to identify expertise have little to no added impact on client outcomes. Additionally, some of the limitations of current traditional training regimes are outlined, along with the emerging evidence base for DP as a training method that can help improve the acquisition of therapeutic skills and expertise.

Keywords: Deliberate practice; psychotherapy outcomes; psychotherapy expertise; psychotherapy training; therapist professional development; improved outcomes

Chapter Learning Outcomes

(1) Examine the principles and processes involved in DP.
(2) Identify how a DP training regime can be developed.

Evidence Based Counselling & Psychotherapy for the 21st Century Practitioner, 135–146

Published under exclusive licence by Emerald Publishing Limited
doi:10.1108/978-1-80455-732-720231011

Introduction

If, as we examined in the first chapter, empirically supported treatments are more effective than other bona fide treatments, would it not be expected for outcomes to have improved across time? Weisz et al. (2019) demonstrate that the mental health field has not improved as measured by client outcomes. Weisz et al. (2019) examined 453 randomised control trials (RCTs) spanning 53 years, involving nearly 32,000 children treated for several psychological and social presenting issues and found that overall outcomes have not improved. At the same time, outcome studies with adults across 'diagnoses' reflect these findings, and aggregated effect sizes have not improved in over four decades (Wampold & Imel, 2015). When we consider this within the context of other research that suggests in general individual practitioners do not get better with time and experience (Chow et al., 2015; Germer, Weyrich, Bräscher, Mütze, & Witthöft, 2022; Goldberg, Babins-Wagner, et al., 2016), it highlights some possible limitations of our current systems of training practitioners and their on-going professional development. Recent innovations in the training and ongoing development of practitioners referred to as DP is one method proposed that can help practitioners develop more effectively by individualising training regimes to meet specific deficits and areas for improvement.

Therapist Training

The literature has historically been somewhat ambiguous when it comes to the professional training of counsellors and psychotherapists. While Garfield and Bergin (1971) found a positive outcome between therapist experience and client outcomes, other research is not so supportive, leading Christensen and Jacobson (1994) to suggest that training doctoral-level practitioner is not justified. Further, Lambert (2015, p. 88) tells us that 'training programs are also highly diverse with little agreement across the world about the type and amount of training necessary for effective practice'. Regarding the level of training, Owen, Wampold, Kopta, Rousmaniere, and Miller (2016) showed that psychotherapy training produces a small-sized growth in therapists' outcomes, however, this was mediated by initial client distress. Said another way, therapists improved slightly with clients who were not as distressed at baseline, however, with more distressed clients, no such improvements were exhibited, irrespective of trainee level. Erekson et al.'s (2017) longitude study found that the magnitude and speed of change produced by established doctoral psychologists did not improve, and in general slowed slightly as they progressed to later training stages. Goldberg, Rousmaniere, et al. (2016) in another longitudinal study of effectiveness demonstrated that practitioners' outcomes diminished slightly over time. In fact, student therapists (Dyason et al., 2020) and paraprofessionals often have client outcomes as good as established professionals. Other research informs us that years practicing, level of qualification, and modality used are not predictive of outcome (Clement, 1994; Germer et al., 2022; Wampold & Brown, 2005), our other great go to for development, personal psychotherapy has also shown not to predict outcomes (Moe & Thimm, 2021).

Anderson, Ogles, Patterson, Lambert, and Vermeersch (2009) contend a well-defined set of facilitative interpersonal skills are what makes practitioners effective, and makes some more effective than others, a contention that would be consistent with the idea of evidence based relationships and responsiveness outlined in this book. As such, and supported by the research set out across previous chapters, learning a new modality or collection of techniques is unlikely to improve your overall effectiveness as a practitioner. Indeed, based on this research, Tracey, Wampold, Lichtenberg, and Goodyear (2014) postulate that the field of psychotherapy is without expertise. However, one method for improving overall effectiveness is by developing an individualised DP plan based on the variables discussed across this book. I say individualised because just choosing where to start without first identifying where one is at is not an efficient or indeed an effective use of time. As such, developing a base line of effectiveness is needed in addition to deliberately practicing and acquiring new skills. Therefore, in this chapter, I will provide an overview of how to support the acquisition of new skills and expertise through DP and in the following chapter, Dr Jeb Brown and I illustrate how using data in supervision is another aspect of DP that provides fruitful areas for practitioners to develop in.

Individual Therapist Effects

Therapist effects (TE) describe the difference between practitioners' ability to effect change, it has nothing to do with the theories and techniques used by practitioners, but it is what they do differently. Therapist effects have come under increased attention, they are still a relatively new area of interest, with less known about how and why they occur. Individual TE account for 5–9% of the outcome variable (Baldwin & Imel, 2013; Firth, Saxon, Stiles, & Barkham, 2019; Wampold & Imel, 2015). Wampold and Brown's (2005) meta-analysis suggests that client gender, age, or diagnosis provided, as well as therapist age, gender, experience, and professional degree accounted for little of the variability in outcomes among therapists. Moreover, individual practitioners produce dropout rates in the range of 1.2–73.2%, while others consistently exhibit practices whereby their clients deteriorate while in their care (Okiishi, Lambert, Nielsen, & Ogles, 2003; Saxon, Firth, & Barkham, 2017). One issue of concern is that practitioners are generally poor at identifying clients not benefiting from therapy (Hannan et al., 2005; Hatfield, McCullough, Frantz, & Krieger, 2010; Lambert, 2013). Indeed, it is proposed that practitioners routinely and vastly overestimate their effectiveness and find it difficult to identify those at risk of poor outcomes (Chow et al., 2015; Hannon et al., 2005).

The most effective practitioners can work with clients presenting with more severe symptomatology and gain better results (Firth et al., 2019; Johns, Barkham, Kellett, & Saxon, 2019; Saxon & Barkham, 2012). Moreover, these highly effective therapists in the top quartile achieve outcomes more than twice that of those in the bottom (Wampold & Brown, 2005). Okiishi et al. (2003, p. 1) demonstrated that 'therapists whose clients showed the fastest rate of improvement had an average rate of change 10 times greater than the mean for the sample. The therapists whose clients showed the slowest rate of improvement exhibited an average increase in symptoms among their clients'. At the same time, therapist effectiveness is not necessarily a global construct and a practitioner with expertise in treating one issue, such as anxiety may not necessarily be effective in treating a different one, such as anxiety with comorbid issues (Kraus, Castonguay, Boswell, Nordberg, & Hayes, 2011; Kraus et al., 2016). Furthermore, therapists vary in their ability to develop the therapeutic alliance, this has major implications when considered in the context of a study by Baldwin, Wampold, and Imel (2007) who found that it was the practitioners' contribution to the alliance that is more important. Thus, with differences of this magnitude across individual therapists, one is justified in calling into question the current training regimes and the standardised competency framework in place. DP offers a method to assist with making improvements in these areas based on individualised therapist needs.

Deliberate Practice

DP has a short history in psychotherapy as an evidence based method of training practitioners in the acquisition of skills and improvement in expertise. However, DP has been around for some time and has a huge body of evidence to support its proposition that it helps practitioners of a variety of fields become superior performers (Ericsson, 2003, 2018). Anders Ericsson is the social psychologist who first referred to a method of training called DP, he postulated:

> Analysing a review of laboratory studies of learning and skill acquisition during the last century, we found that improvement of performance was uniformly observed when people were given tasks with well-defined goals, were provided with feedback, and had ample opportunities for repetition. These deliberate efforts to increase one's performance beyond its current level involve problem solving and finding better methods to perform the tasks. When a person engages in a practice activity (typically designed by teachers) with the primary goal of improving some aspect of performance, we called that activity deliberate practice. (p. 67)

DP, and DP research, with regard to psychotherapy is still in its infancy. However, the quest for better results and the development of expertise has been linked to DP by several researchers (Anderson & Perlman, 2020; Miller, Hubble, & Chow, 2020; Rousmaniere, Goodyear, Miller, & Wampold, 2017; Wampold, Lichtenberg, Goodyear, & Tracey, 2019). DP contains five processes that are not present in regular therapy training, or continuous professional development:

(1) Setting learning goals just beyond your ability.
(2) Getting expert feedback from a coach/consultant.
(3) Repetitive behavioural rehearsal of specific skills.
(4) Observing your work.
(5) Continuously assessing performance.

We can see these five processes in the definition provided by Ericsson and Pool (2016, p. 157) when they suggest that the distinctive feature of DP

> is that you try to do something you cannot do – that takes you out of your comfort zone – and that you practice it over and over again focusing on exactly how you are doing it, where you are falling short, and how you can get better.

Before I unpack DP further, several key studies from the extant literature are discussed.

In a seminal study of DP, Chow et al. (2015, p. 337) demonstrated that the amount of time spent targeting therapist skill was predictive of client outcome, with those spending more time reviewing recordings of session being most effective. Similarly, Goldberg, Rousmaniere, et al. (2016) examined a whole agency (153 practitioners and 5,128 clients) engaged in DP with findings suggesting that small gains were made within practitioners' caseloads each year across the seven years of the study. Of course, these are two relatively small studies, methodologically speaking, and more research needs to be carried out, but all the indications are indicative of DP being an innovative training regime. While the previous DP studies that I have mentioned take a more macro analysis of DP effectiveness, with regard to client outcomes, other studies examine DP in the acquisition of skills and expertise across a broad range of therapeutic variables in training workshops (e.g. Anderson, Perlman, McCarrick, & McClintock, 2020; Barrett-Naylor et al., 2020; Di Bartolomeo, Shukla, Westra, Shekarak Ghashghaei, & Olson, 2021; McLeod, 2021; Perlman, Anderson, Foley, Mimnaugh, & Safran, 2020; Westra et al., 2021).

Newman et al. (2022) provide evidence that DP is helpful for psychologists to build communication skills during the consultation process, while McLeod (2021) demonstrated that students in counsellor training found DP beneficial for learning a range of counselling skills, although it took time for the students to internalise the DP framework. DP has been put forward as a training method to assist practitioners work with client resistance, with Westra et al. (2021) demonstrating that a DP workshop can enhance trainees' responsiveness to working with resistance. Participants in this study reported satisfaction with the DP method and were rated as demonstrating more skills on all measures post workshop when compared against the control group. In a similar study examining resistance with the use of motivational interviewing, Di Bartolomeo et al. (2021) found that when compared against traditional methods of training practitioners in the use of motivational interviewing, that those in the DP group elicited less resistance.

In a study seeking to improve the immediacy skills of psychologists, Hill et al. (2020) found that DP helped practitioners become aware of and manage feelings and counter-transference that stopped them from using immediacy. Two other DP studies address facilitative interpersonal skills and the therapeutic alliance. Perlman et al. (2020) found that participants in the DP group had 'significantly higher levels of specifically targeted post-training therapist skills such as, empathy, alliance bond capacity, and alliance rupture-repair responsiveness' compared against traditional methods of training. Moreover, Anderson et al. (2020) demonstrated that skill acquisition can be enhanced using DP drills for facilitative interpersonal skills. While there still needs to be much more research on DP, research indicates that this is a valid and promising method for practitioners to enhance their development. DP is not just a valuable method for the initial training of practitioners, ongoing development through continuous professional education can also benefit from DP, this is essential considering some of the findings that ongoing development activities such as reading and attending workshops don't generally improve practitioners' effectiveness (Taylor & Neimeyer, 2017).

What DP Is, and Is Not

As DP is still in its infancy, there has been some confusion as to what it is, and more importantly, what it is not. Thus, for research and practice to move forward, DP needs to be conceptualised clearly. Vaz and Rousmaniere (2021) provide five areas of clarification that distinguishes DP from traditional methods. For example, one of the differentiating factors between DP and other methods is the focus on procedural over conceptual learning. Traditional conceptual training involves attending lectures and reading academic texts, note taking, and watching the practice of simulated therapy sessions. While these are all important elements of practitioner training, and can occur in conjunction with DP, they are primarily intellectual activities and they are not procedural learning methods. Procedural practice involves the repeated rehearsal of specific skills, with immediate feedback from a more knowledgeable other (MKO), with the specific skills further refined based on feedback.

Critically, for practitioners, this behavioural rehearsal happens outside of the therapeutic hour in the same way as a musician or sports player will practice before a concert or sports match. While both the musician and sports player must learn how their respective fields of interest work (conceptual), they must put this into practice by identifying areas for skills acquisition (procedural).

So, what does DP look like operationalised and how does this method differ from regular training that seeks to develop therapeutic skills. Firstly, in traditional training or continued professional education, skills training tends to be delivered at the whole group/class level as opposed to the individualised methods of DP. Thus, learners are not identifying individual learning goals just beyond their ability. Secondly, in traditional training while there is a rehearsal of clinical skills training through a dialogue with a trainee playing the role of a 'practitioner' and another taking on the role of the 'client', this tends to be a free-flowing dialogue where the 'practitioner' tracks the 'client's' story, shifting and attempting to intervene with different clinical skills at certain points in the process as the story evolves. Another point to note, is that while there may be some reflection afterwards with a MKO, or indeed a peer, this self-reflection tends to be performance based with strengths and weaknesses identified, and in some cases more appropriate therapy skills modelled by the MKO without the practitioner rehearsing these skills repetitively.

Although the above are certainly valuable to the new and more experienced practitioner, it is not DP. This traditional method lacks repetition and successive refinement, in addition to the training often having a standardised focus. In contrast, Ericsson and Lehmann (1996, p. 278) clearly define DP as 'the individualized training activities specially designed by a coach or teacher to improve specific aspects of an individual's performance through repetition and successive refinement'. So, drawing on the five processes of DP identified previously, I will outline how a practitioner can use DP to improve skills acquisition while learning empathy.

(1) Setting learning goals just beyond your current ability:
John, a practitioner, has been attending supervision with a new supervisor who likes to use DP when possible. As John has gone back to study for his doctorate having been a practicing therapist for many years, the supervisor thought that it would be a good opportunity to use DP due to the training course mandating John to audio record session for developmental purposes. Upon listening to several tapes, John's supervisor notices that John expresses empathetic understanding at about a level 2 (You will recall the five levels from previous chapter). John agrees with the supervisor that he would like to improve his empathy and the supervisor devises an individualised DP training for John.
The training requires john to respond empathetically to a simulated client video. The DP exercise is based on responding to first to explicit emption, followed by implicit emotion in the context of the clients two minute video.

(2) Getting expert feedback from a coach:
The supervisor plays the simulated client video and John responds based on the two criteria, explicit, then implicit emotion. The supervisor (MKO) then provides John with feedback based on his response, and guides him on how it can be approved upon.

(3) Repetitive behavioural rehearsal of specific skills:
John continues to practice his response, with successive refining when needed based on the continuous feedback from the supervisor. Critically, John is responding to the same stimulus in the simulated video and using the same two criteria each time in order to provide a consistent way to assess and improve performance.

(4) Observing your work:
Many people who use DP to develop expertise either video record or audio record actual therapy session and bring these recordings to supervision, and/or watch them back in their own time to identify areas to improve on. This means that the practitioner can develop these skills outside of formal supervision as this is where most of the DP effort needs to be directed. We are not practicing when we are actually in a real therapy session, we are preforming. So, just like the sports player, there needs to be practice and training outside of these official times which can help build capacity for actual therapy sessions. John continues to watch himself back on the tapes and brings them to supervision for feedback.

(5) Continuously assessing performance:
Assessing performance is a little bit more tricky as it brings us into the domain of developing a baselines of effectiveness in more objective ways (discussed in the next chapter). However, along with a coach or supervisor, progress on the acquisition of these skills can be assessed on an ongoing basis by watching back recording of DP exercises, or indeed real therapy sessions. Progress can then be tracked through mining outcome data.

Where to Direct DP Efforts

DP takes time and effort to see results from. Therefore, directing your efforts needs to be done thoughtfully and with purpose. For me, targeting the big impact variables discussed in the previous chapters is possibly the best place to start (if you don't have data to base this decision on), the practitioner who needs to improve empathy will gain more from this than from learning the next new technique that will add little to improving the overall effectiveness of the practitioner. Of course, some practitioners may very well have refined empathy skills and learning to become more proficient in another of the variables will be beneficial. Thus, I come back to my point from earlier, that individualised DP is what is needed, leading me to suggest that practitioners willing to undertake a DP training regime should in the first instance assess themselves against the variables outlined in this book. While I agree with Miller et al. (2020) that there is relatively little difference in therapy models and as such the use of DP to improve outcomes should focus on the common factor big variables, there is still milage to be had in using DP to learn new, or improve existing techniques, especially where deficiencies have been identified. In addition, I believe that DP can be helpful, especially for models that seek to provide a cogent rationale, to provide structure and to build expectancy of positive outcomes, as discussed in earlier chapters. As such, my thinking on this reflects that of Vaz and Rousmaniere (2021, p. 67) who summarise this debate eloquently:

> The fact is that therapists are more likely to intervene in an authentic, verbally fluent and persuasive manner if they do so in association with one or more theoretical frameworks that they personally value and identify with. What does this mean, pragmatically, for DP in psychotherapy? That therapists should learn to acquire a sense of confidence and mastery over skills and models they believe in, while also keeping a close eye on the impact of said skills on the therapeutic alliance and client outcomes.

Conclusion

DP is an emerging innovative method for the initial training of practitioners, and seasoned practitioners' ongoing professional development. Research exposes to us that many of the criteria that we use to establish effectiveness and professionalism may not actually impact on client outcomes. Years practicing, level of qualification, modality used, gender accreditation/licensure on ongoing continuing professional development training do not seem to improve a practitioners overall effectiveness after initial training, and indeed in some cases while still in training. DP linked to high impact variables discussed in this book is one place for the practitioner to begin their DP training regime, with the support of an MKO. Practitioners must find their sweet spot in order to stretch their capacity, just like Goldilocks it must be not too hot, or not to cold. Said another way, practitioners must find their individual zone of proximity in order to develop through DP. Finally, no matter the DP regime a practitioner enters into, they should expect to see improvements in their effectiveness as demonstrated by improved client outcomes. In order to demonstrate this, there needs to be some method of assessing and tracking how the practitioner is developing objectively. The next chapter examines the use of data to do this, while it can also be used to inform DP in the supervisory space.

References

Anderson, T., Ogles, B. M., Patterson, C. L., Lambert, M. J., & Vermeersch, D. A. (2009). Therapist effects: Facilitative interpersonal skills as a predictor of therapist success. *Journal of Clinical Psychology*, *65*, 755–768. https://doi.org/10.1002/jclp.20583

Anderson, T., & Perlman, M. R. (2020). Therapeutic interpersonal skills for facilitating the working alliance. In J. N. Fuertes (Ed.), *Working alliance skills for mental health professionals* (pp. 43–68). New York, NY: Oxford.

Anderson, T., Perlman, M. R., McCarrick, S. M., & McClintock, A. S. (2020). Modeling therapist responses with structured practice enhances facilitative interpersonal skills. *Journal of Clinical Psychology*, *76*(4), 659–675.

Baldwin, S. A., & Imel, Z. E. (2013). Therapist effects: Findings and methods. In M. J. Lambert (Ed.), *Bergin and Garfield's handbook of psychotherapy and behavior change* (6th ed., pp. 259–297). Hoboken, NJ: Wiley.

Baldwin, S. A., Wampold, B. E., & Imel, Z. E. (2007). Untangling the alliance-outcome correlation: Exploring the relative importance of therapist and patient variability in the alliance. *Journal of Consulting and Clinical Psychology*, *75*(6), 842–852. https://doi.org/10.1037/0022-006X.75.6.842

Barrett-Naylor, R., Malins, S., Levene, J., Biswas, S., Mays, C., & Main, G. (2020). Brie training in psychological assessment and interventions skills for cancer care staff: A mixed methods evaluation of deliberate practice techniques. *Psycho-Oncology*, *29*(11), 1786–1793.

Chow, D. L., Miller, S. D., Seidel, J. A., Kane, R. T., Thornton, J. A., & Andrews, W. P. (2015). The role of deliberate practice in the development of highly effective psychotherapists. *Psychotherapy*, *52*(3), 337–345. https://doi.org/10.1037/pst0000015

Christensen, A., & Jacobson, N. S. (1994). Who (or what) can do psychotherapy: The status and challenge of nonprofessional therapies. *Psychological Science*, *5*(1), 8–14. https://doi.org/10.1111/j.1467-9280.1994.tb00606.x

Clement, P. W. (1994). Quantitative evaluation of 26 years of private practice. *Professional Psychology: Research and Practice*, *25*(2), 173–176. https://doi.org/10.1037/0735-7028.25.2.173

Di Bartolomeo, A. A., Shukla, S., Westra, H. A., Shekarak Ghashghaei, N., & Olson, D. A. (2021). Rolling with resistance: A client language analysis of deliberate practice in continuing education for psychotherapists. *Counselling and Psychotherapy Research*, *21*, 434–442. https://doi.org/10.1002/capr.12335

Dyason, K. M., Shanley, D. C., O'Donovan, A., & Low-Choy, S. (2020). Does feedback improve psychotherapy outcomes compared to treatment-as-usual for adults and youth?. *Psychotherapy Research*, *30*(3), 310–324.

Ericsson, K. A. (2003). The acquisition of expert performance as problem solving: Construction and modification of mediating mechanisms through deliberate practice. In J. E. Davidson & R. J. Sternberg (Eds.), *The psychology of problem solving* (pp. 31–83). Cambridge: Cambridge University Press. https://doi.org/10.1017/CBO9780511615771.003

Ericsson, K. A. (2018). The differential influence of experience, practice, and deliberate practice on the development of superior individual performance of experts. In K. A. Ericsson, R. R. Hoffman, A. Kozbelt, & A. M. Williams (Eds.), *The Cambridge handbook of expertise and expert performance* (pp. 745–769). Cambridge: Cambridge University Press.

Ericsson, K. A., & Lehmann, A. C. (1996). Expert and exceptional performance: evidence of maximal adaptation to task constraints. *Annual Review of Psychology*, *47*, 273–305. https://doi.org/10.1146/annurev.psych.47.1.273

Ericsson, A., & Pool, R. (2016). *Peak: Secrets from the new science of expertise*. San Francisco, CA: Houghton Mifflin Harcourt.

Erekson, D. M., Janis, R., Bailey, R. J., Cattani, K., & Pedersen, T. R. (2017). A longitudinal investigation of the impact of psychotherapist training: Does training improve client outcomes? *Journal of Counseling Psychology*, *64*(5), 514–524. https://doi.org/10.1037/cou0000252

Firth, N., Saxon, D., Stiles, W. B., & Barkham, M. (2019). Therapist and clinic effects in psychotherapy: A three-level model of outcome variability. *Journal of Consulting and Clinical Psychology*, *87*(4), 345–356. https://doi.org/10.1037/ccp0000388

Garfield, S. L., & Bergin, A. E. (1971). Personal therapy, outcome and some therapist variables. *Psychotherapy: Theory, Research & Practice*, *8*(3), 251–253. https://doi.org/10.1037/h0086667

Germer, S., Weyrich, V., Bräscher, A. K., Mütze, K., & Witthöft, M. (2022). Does practice really make perfect? A longitudinal analysis of the relationship between therapist experience and therapy outcome: A replication of Goldberg, Rousmaniere, et al. (2016). *Journal of Counseling Psychology*. Advance online publication. https://doi.org/10.1037/cou0000608

Goldberg, S. B., Babins-Wagner, R., Rousmaniere, T., Berzins, S., Hoyt, W. T., Whipple, J. L., … Wampold, B. E. (2016). Creating a climate for therapist improvement: A case study of an agency focused on outcomes and deliberate practice. *Psychotherapy*, *53*(3), 367–375. https://doi.org/10.1037/pst0000060

Goldberg, S. B., Rousmaniere, T., Miller, S. D., Whipple, J., Nielsen, S. L., Hoyt, W. T., & Wampold, B. E. (2016). Do psychotherapists improve with time and experience? A longitudinal analysis of outcomes in a clinical setting. *Journal of Counseling Psychology*, *63*(1), 1–11. https://doi.org/10.1037/cou0000131

Hannan, C., Lambert, M. J., Harmon, C., Nielsen, S. L., Smart, D. W., Shimokawa, K., & Sutton, S. W. (2005). A lab test and algorithms for identifying clients at risk for treatment failure. *Journal of Clinical Psychology*, *61*(2), 155–163. https://doi.org/10.1002/jclp.20108

Hatfield, D., McCullough, L., Frantz, S. H., & Krieger, K. (2010). Do we know when our clients get worse? An investigation of therapists' ability to detect negative client change. *Clinical Psychology & Psychotherapy*, *17*(1), 25–32. https://doi.org/10.1002/cpp.656

Hill, C. E., Kivlighan, D. M., III, Rousmaniere, T., Kivlighan, D. M., Jr, Gerstenblith, J. A., & Hillman, J. W. (2020). Deliberate practice for the skill of immediacy: A multiple case study of doctoral student therapists and clients. *Psychotherapy*, *57*(4), 587–597. https://doi.org/10.1037/pst0000247

Johns, R. G., Barkham, M., Kellett, S., & Saxon, D. (2019). A systematic review of therapist effects: A critical narrative update and refinement to review. *Clinical Psychology Review*, *67*, 78–93. https://doi.org/10.1016/j.cpr.2018.08.004

Kraus, D., Castonguay, L., Boswell, J., Nordberg, S., & Hayes, J. A. (2011). Therapist effectiveness: Implications for accountability and patient care. *Psychotherapy Research*, *21*(3), 267–276. doi:10.1080/10503307.2011.563249

Kraus, D. R., Bentley, J. H., Alexander, P. C., Boswell, J. F., Constantino, M. J., Baxter, E. E., & Castonguay, L. G. (2016). Predicting therapist effectiveness from their own practice-based evidence. *Journal of Consulting and Clinical Psychology*, *84*(6), 473–483. https://doi.org/10.1037/ccp0000083

Lambert, M. (2015). Effectiveness of psychotherapeutic treatment. *Resonances – E-Journal for Biopsychosocial Dialogues in Psychosomatic Medicine, Psychotherapy, Supervision and Counseling*, *3*(2), 87–100. Retrieved from https://www.resonanzen-journal.org/index.php/resonanzen/article/view/373. Accessed on June 8, 2022.

Lambert, M. J. (2013). Outcome in psychotherapy: The past and important advances. *Psychotherapy*, *50*(1), 42–51. https://doi.org/10.1037/a0030682

McLeod, J. (2021). How students use deliberate practice during the first stage of counsellor training. *Counselling and Psychotherapy Research*, *22*, 207–218. https://doi.org/10.1002/capr.12397

Miller, S. D., Hubble, M. A., & Chow, D. (2020). *Better results: Using deliberate practice to improve therapeutic effectiveness*. Washington, DC: American Psychological Association.

Moe, F. D., & Thimm, J. (2021). Personal therapy and the personal therapist. *Nordic Psychology*, *73*(1), 3–28. doi:10.1080/19012276.2020.1762713

Newman, D. S., Villarreal, J. N., Gerrard, M. K., McIntire, H., Barrett, C. A., & Kaiser, L. T. (2022). Deliberate practice of consultation communication skills: A randomized controlled trial. *School Psychology*, *37*(3), 225–235. https://doi.org/10.1037/spq0000494

Okiishi, J., Lambert, M. J., Nielsen, S. L., & Ogles, B. M. (2003). Waiting for supershrink: An empirical analysis of therapist effects. *Clinical Psychology & Psychotherapy*, *10*, 361–373. https://doi.org/10.1002/cpp.383

Owen, J., Wampold, B. E., Kopta, M., Rousmaniere, T., & Miller, S. D. (2016). As good as it gets? Therapy outcomes of trainees over time. *Journal of Counseling Psychology*, *63*(1), 12–19. https://doi.org/10.1037/cou0000112

Perlman, M. R., Anderson, T., Foley, V. K., Mimnaugh, S., & Safran, J. D. (2020). The impact of alliance-focused and facilitative interpersonal relationship training on therapist skills: An RCT of brief training. *Psychotherapy Research*, *30*(7), 871–884.

Rousmaniere, T., Goodyear, R. K., Miller, S. D., & Wampold, B. E. (Eds.). (2017). *The cycle of excellence: Using deliberate practice to improve supervision and training*. Hoboken, NJ: John Wiley & Sons.

Saxon, D., & Barkham, M. (2012). Patterns of therapist variability: Therapist effects and the contribution of patient severity and risk. *Journal of Consulting and Clinical Psychology*, *80*(4), 535–546. https://doi.org/10.1037/a0028898

Saxon, D., Firth, N., & Barkham, M. (2017). The relationship between therapist effects and therapy delivery factors: Therapy modality, dosage, and non-completion. *Administration and Policy in Mental Health and Mental Health Services Research*, *44*, 705–715. https://doi.org/10.1007/s10488-016-0750-5

Taylor, J. M., & Neimeyer, G. J. (2017). Continuing education and lifelong learning strategies. In S. Walfish, J. E. Barnett, & J. Zimmerman (Eds.), *Handbook of private practice: Keys to success for mental health practitioners* (pp. 602–618). Oxford: Oxford University Press. https://doi.org/10.1093/med:psych/9780190272166.003.0046

Tracey, T., Wampold, B. E., Lichtenberg, J. W., & Goodyear, R. K. (2014). Expertise in psychotherapy: An elusive goal? *American Psychologist*, *69*(3), 218–229. https://doi.org/10.1037/a0035099

Vaz, A., & Rousmaniere, T. (2021). *Reaching for expertise: A primer on deliberate practice for psychotherapists*. Seattle, WA: Sentio University.

Wampold, B. E., & Brown, G. S. (J.). (2005). Estimating variability in outcomes attributable to therapists: A naturalistic study of outcomes in managed care. *Journal of Consulting and Clinical Psychology*, *73*(5), 914–923. https://doi.org/10.1037/0022-006X.73.5.914

Wampold, B. E., & Imel, Z. E. (2015). *The great psychotherapy debate* (2nd ed.). New York, NY: Routledge/Taylor & Francis Group.

Wampold, B. E., Lichtenberg, J. W., Goodyear, R. K., & Tracey, T. J. (2019). Clinical expertise. In S. Dimidjian (Ed.), *Evidence-based practice in action: Bridging clinical science and intervention* (pp. 152–166). New York, NY: Guilford Publications.

Weisz, J. R., Kuppens, S., Ng, M. Y., Vaughn-Coaxum, R. A., Ugueto, A. M., Eckshtain, D., & Corteselli, K. A. (2019). Are psychotherapies for young people growing stronger? Tracking trends over time for youth anxiety, depression, attention-deficit/hyperactivity disorder, and conduct problems. *Perspectives on Psychological Science: A Journal of the Association for Psychological Science*, *14*(2), 216–237. https://doi.org/10.1177/1745691618805436

Westra, H. A., Norouzian, N., Poulin, L., Coyne, A., Constantino, M. J., Hara, K., … Antony, M. M. (2021). Testing a deliberate practice workshop for developing appropriate responsivity to resistance markers. *Psychotherapy*, *58*(2), 175–185. https://doi.org/10.1037/pst0000311

Chapter 12

Enhancing Supervision Through the Use of Data

Daryl Mahon and Jeb Brown

Abstract

Supervision is considered the signature pedagogy and after direct client practice it is rated as the number one learning and development method by practitioners. However, as we set out in this chapter, the relationship between supervision and client outcomes is not a strong one. Drawing on the use of routine outcome data, we demonstrate how clinical supervision can be improved when both practitioner and supervisor demonstrate an attitude of humility and a willingness to learn from the data they collect. Using these data to enhance supervision by improving client outcomes and to inform deliberate practice (DP) is the hall mark of the effective twenty-first century practitioner and supervisor.

Keywords: Supervision; deliberate practice; data-informed supervision; continuous professional development; psychotherapy outcomes; outcome monitoring

Chapter Learning Outcomes

(1) Understand how supervision can be improved by using outcome data.
(2) Explore how supervision and data can contribute to DP.

Introduction

Watkins (2020) considers supervision the key signature pedagogies of psychiatry and other related mental health professions such as psychology and

Evidence Based Counselling & Psychotherapy for the 21st Century Practitioner, 147–157

Published under exclusive licence by Emerald Publishing Limited
doi:10.1108/978-1-80455-732-720231012

counselling. Although several definitions of supervision are in the literature, they often share similar themes and functions. Specifically, supervision is described as a learning and development endeavour, provided by a more senior person of similar profession. Supervision is a reflective and developmental environment, relationship focussed, and focusses on the accusation of skills, knowledge, and competencies. Supervision has as a main concern ethically sound work, the achievement of organisational goals, and that the supervisees wellbeing needs are met (Hawkins & Shoet, 2012; Morrison, 2005; Watkins, 2020). Bernard and Goodyear (1992, p. 8) provide the following definition of clinical supervision: 'this relationship is evaluative, extends over time and has the simultaneous purposes of enhancing the professional functioning of the more junior person and monitoring the quality of the professional'. Of course, supervisors and supervisees believe in the benefits, power, and efficacy of supervision (Rast, Herman, Rousmaniere, Whipple, & Swift, 2017). Yet, belief does not necessarily mean an empirical reality, at least as far as client outcomes are concerned. Most certainly supervision has a host of benefits for the practitioner: emotional support, reflective practice, ethical decision making among them. However, it is argued in this chapter, and indeed in the literature, that the yardstick to measure the value of supervision should be in the ability of the supervisory dyad to improve client outcomes.

Impact of Supervision on Outcomes

Wrape, Callahan, Ruggero, and Watkins (2015, p. 36) posit that the criteria by which to evaluate supervision's efficacy lies in its power to bring about favourable client changes. Watkins (2020) reviewing the supervision research literature across the last 25 years suggests that "evidence based supervision appears more a hope and dream than an evidence based reality. Moreover, Watkins suggests that supervision models generally lack empirical foundation and evidence supporting supervision impact of any type is weak at best, especially so for practitioner and client outcomes. Snowdon, Leggat, and Taylor's (2017) systematic review found that there was no correlation between supervision and client experience. For Carpenter, Webb, and Bostock (2013), much like Watkins (2011, 2020), the most obvious gap is in evidence that models of supervision lead to improved outcomes for workers and clients of practitioners. Kühne, Maas, Wiesenthal, and Weck (2019) in a systematic review found that supervision appears to be seen as helpful by supervisees. In another systematic review, Alfonsson, Parling, Spännargård, Andersson, and Lundgren (2018) found that supervision may benefit novice practitioner's competency but reflecting previous studies has no evidence of impact on client outcomes. Likewise, Bogo and McKnight (2006) and Carpenter et al. (2013) draw similar conclusions, contending that supervision's positive impact on practitioner outcomes is weak at best.

Supervisors explained less than 1% of the variance in client psychotherapy outcomes in a study of 175 therapists with five years of data (Rousmaniere, Swift, Babins-Wagner, Whipple, & Berzins, 2016). In a replication study, Whipple et al. (2020) examined the amount of variance in client outcome that is attributable to supervision, based on a longitudinal dataset of 3,030 clients, 80 therapists, and 39 supervisors. Similarly, to the Rousmaniere et al. (2016) study, they found that supervisors accounted for 0% of the variance in client outcome. Both studies had one to two hours per week of individual supervision, with the Rousmaniere et al. (2016) study having two-hour weekly group supervision, in addition to individual supervision.

Using Feedback Data in Supervision

There is a relative dearth of research exploring the use of client feedback in the supervisory relationship, and what studies there are, contain small samples. Bambling, King, Raue, Schweitzer, and Lambert (2006) compared a supervision group of practitioners to inactive controls, the supervision group when taught to focus on alliance process and monitor client feedback, resulted in the supervision group doing better than the control group across factors and processes such as working alliance, symptom reduction, and treatment retention. At the same time, Grossl, Reese, Norsworthy, and Hopkins (2014) report that practitioners who used client feedback data during supervision reported greater satisfaction with supervision. Reese et al. (2009) demonstrated that practitioners who discussed their data with supervisors improved more than the control group, and the relationship between self-efficacy and outcome was stronger. Worthen and Lambert (2007) suggest incorporating an outcome management system into supervision in order to help actualise the goals of supervision. One study of note, although not exclusive to the use of feedback alone, demonstrated that when feedback systems are utilised as a part of DP, therapists improve outcomes at a small be meaningful d=0.034 each year (Goldberg et al., 2016). Worthen and Lambert (2007, p. 186) inform us that the use of continuous client outcome data during the supervision process may help to provide the practitioner with the specific feedback he or she desires and finds helpful. However, in this chapter, we seek to go beyond the idea being helpful to promise a model for twenty-first century supervision that includes the use outcome data and DP to measure the improvement of the supervisee's outcomes.

Part of the goal of this chapter is to help supervisors learn to train effective practitioners without presuming that the supervisor must have better outcomes than the supervisee. It was Wampold, Kim, and Bolt (2006) who posed the question 'What characterizes the psychotherapy provided by psychotherapists who consistently get better outcomes and how can we all adopt such practices to improve our effectiveness?' They proposed a three key components of practitioner expertise:

- Focussing on ensuring engagement in the psychotherapy process.
- Attending to the working alliance by focussing on the collaborative nature of our work.
- Receiving feedback about our effectiveness by measuring outcomes.

To further quote from his article:

Garrison Keillor observes of the residents of Lake Wobegon, 'All the women are strong, all the men are good-looking, and all the children are above average'. As psychotherapists, it is likely that we similarly believe we are above average, but as Keillor's folksy humour reminds us, it isn't so – half of us are below average, as a statistical necessity!

Increasingly, the measure of practitioner expertise will be the ability to improve outcomes rather than type of training and years of experience (Tracy et al., 2014, 2015). We need to face the fact that measuring outcomes as a routine part of training and supervision presents new challenges for supervisors. There is no reason to believe that supervisors' outcomes have a significantly different distribution than their supervisees. About half of the supervisors have above average results, as will about half of their supervisees. This assumes a large enough sample that the expected distribution holds. However, in smaller samples, as is often the case, the supervisor distribution of outcomes might be significantly different than the supervisees. For example, imagine being a supervisor in a university counselling centre-based training where researchers analysed several years of archival data on repeated measures of an outcome questionnaire (Minami et al., 2009). The average effect size for the entire clinic was 0.85, which is quite good, well into the highly effective range. Even better, the average effect size for the interns (61 practitioners treating 312 clients) was 1. The effect size of other trainings (41 practitioners treating 85 clients) was 0.92. Excellent!

Of course, there is a catch here. Supervisees have outcomes well above the clinic average which means that you also learnt that the average effect size for the professional staff which includes you (30 practitioners treating 481 patients), had an average effect size of only 0.54, well below the threshold 0.8 effect size to characterise the services as highly effective. Now what do you do?

Skillset and Knowledge Base for the Supervisor

The traditional concept of supervisor or coach assumes that the supervisor is a more knowledgeable other (MKO) capable of providing feedback and coaching that will enhance the performance of the supervisee. As we have seen, there is no reason to believe that the MKO in psychotherapy supervision has better treatment outcomes. So more knowledgeable cannot easily be defined as more effective as a practitioner.

So how should we define the MKO for psychotherapy supervision? The tradition skillsets and knowledge base still apply.

- Internal knowledge acquisition – case conceptualisation, method of treatment, etc.
- Increase range of techniques (behaviours) available to the practitioner in the session.
- Using alliance measure to elicit honest feedback and addressing disruptions in alliance.
- Successfully engage the client in treatment in terms of duration of treatment.
- Successfully engage clients in the chosen method (work) of therapy.

In addition, the supervisor needs the knowledge and skillsets to incorporate the use of data and algorithm-driven feedback inherent to the evidence based practice of routine measurement and feedback.

- *Understanding of basic measurement concepts*
  - o including validity (necessary for choosing measures appropriate for the population);
  - o basic understanding of statistics used in evaluating outcomes (mean, standard deviation, and effect size); and
  - o basic understanding of measurement error and confidence intervals.
- *Measure and understanding personal results:*
  - o It is not necessary to be above average to be effective.
  - o Monitor results over time, including over the course of a career to continuously look for opportunities to improve.
  - o If you aren't measuring, you don't know if you are improving.
- *Administering questionnaires and eliciting honest responses:*
  - o Explain reasons for and importance of the use of questionnaires.
  - o Encourage honesty on both symptom ratings and, in particular, alliance rating.
  - o Praise and encourage alliance ratings that are less than perfect, with the understanding the practitioner is rarely perfect and the feedback is important for treatment success.
  - o Use the questionnaire (including specific items) to look for information the practitioner may not have been aware of.
- *Discussing results with patients:*
  - o Review progress and discuss plans for termination if outcomes are acceptable.
  - o Discuss lack of improvement where necessary to provide encouragement and discuss possible changes in treatment approach based on client feedback.

The task of the supervisor is to transfer this knowledge and enhance the skillsets of the supervisee. We do not need to assume that the supervisor has better treatment outcomes any more than we need to assume that a coach is (or was) a better athlete than his or her players. These are two different sets of skills. While one skillset might arguably enhance the other, there are many examples of great athletes that failed as coaches, and outstanding coaches who were mediocre athletes, though it probably helps if they at least played the sport.

Using Data to Support DP

DP, by its nature, is most effective when immediate objective data-based performance feedback is available. Subjective judgement of improvement can be misleading. Increased confidence does not necessarily correlate with increased effectiveness. In fact, it is possible that the opposite is true (Davis & Curthbert, 2016; Hook, Watkins, Davis, & Owen, 2015; Nissen-Lie, 2020). Can DP measurably improve outcomes? Probably so, particularly if the practitioner hones the basics of establishing rapport and alliance, working with the client to conceptualise the problem and formulate an approach to solve the problem, monitoring improvement, and utilising feedback on alliance.

- How does the practitioner present the questionnaires and explain the importance of their use?
- How does the practitioner work with the client to establish the basics of working alliance?
    - o Agreement on the nature of the problem.
    - o Agreement on the approach to solving the problem.
    - o Establishment of a trusting relationship based on empathy, compassion, and honesty.
- How does the practitioner encourage honesty in feedback, particularly on the alliance items?
- How does the practitioner address feedback on alliance or rupture in alliance?
- How does the practitioner monitor their data and look for clues they might have missed?

There is a good chance that a practitioner honing these basic skills will find that their outcomes improve over time (Brown, Cazauvieilh, & Simon, 2021; Brown, Simon, & Foster, 2021; Mahon, Brown, & Simon, 2021a, 2021b). All these skills lend themselves to practice in terms of preferred scripts and behaviours. Use of video monitoring and review of behavioural performance of the skill being practiced is ideal, while audio recording is also useful. The lack of any ability to review the behaviours being practiced is a certain impediment to the use of DP.

Drilling down to more granular levels of DP to improve results from specific types of problems is more challenging, but worth pursuing once a practitioner masters the basics. While it is certainly difficult to demonstrate statistically significant improvement in results for subgroups of clients, this does not mean that finding areas for incremental improvement won't translate into overall effectiveness. A practitioner who is data informed can look for clues in their data for learning opportunities.

- Learning from cases with poor outcomes. What might have been done differently?
- Learning what types of challenges the clients might present for that practitioner:
    - o Narcissistic
    - o Highly emotion
    - o Suicidal
    - o Severely depressed
    - o Extremely anxious
    - o Dependent
    - o Aggressive
    - o Substance use.

Arguably all the different ways that clients manifest their problems when entering treatment require different specific skillsets or repertoires of well-practiced behaviours. While the basics account for much of the improvement, the practitioner's ability to adjust his or her verbal and physical behaviours flexibly to meet the highly varied needs of the client both as they present to treatment, and through their response to treatment varies over time. While the net gain in global outcomes may be relatively small, when one is seeking to improve performance, every incremental gain counts!

Cultivating an Attitude of Humility, Curiosity, and the Search for Improvement

In contrast to the goal of creating confidence in expertise, the supervisor models the humility and curiosity needed to improve performance. What does this mean in the context of supervision? Discovering that one's outcomes are below average perhaps helps to eliminate over confidence. There is certainly room for improvement, and some anxiety can be a powerful motivator. Research on decision making and expert judgement reveals that experts in many fields are subject to common human errors that arise from heuristics and cognitive biases (Kahneman, 2011). One of the implications is that there is a risk in becoming too dependent on theories of psychopathology and therapy. The ability to explore and appreciate the uniqueness of the client's experience and presentation in therapy, not to mention the client's own theory of change, may be impaired.

The routine use of questionnaires provides the practitioner the opportunities to look for clues that might otherwise have missed. Explaining to the client that the questionnaires will help the practitioner to do a better job, and that honesty is important, communicates to the client an openness and curiosity while downplaying the wisdom and expertise of the therapist. Humility in action. Humility need not imply lack of confidence in the client's ability to change. The practitioner can certainly convey an attitude of positive expectations and hope because in fact most clients experience improvement regardless of the overall effectiveness of the practitioner. Practitioner humility can also enhance the client's sense of self-efficacy rather than attributing their improvement to the expertise of the practitioner. An attitude of humility and curiosity is also useful even if the practitioner's outcomes are well above average. While increasing outcomes for practitioners in the upper quartile of the effect size distribution may require more focussed effort, and the gains may be incremental, this is true in virtually every domain of expertise and performance. Rather than being self-satisfied, the true modern expert constantly looks for opportunities to improve performance.

Using Feedback to Improve Supervision

The relationship in supervision has been found to be an important variable to consider in effective supervision (Grossl et al., 2014). Specifically, Ellis (1991) found that supervisees rated the relationship with their supervisor as the most important factor in positive supervision. In addition, the supervisory alliance has been found to be correlated with supervision satisfaction and practitioner self-efficacy (Reese et al., 2009; Son & Ellis, 2013). Nelson, Barnes, Evans, and

Triggiano (2008) found that supervisors who were rated very highly by supervisees had characteristics such as openness to conflict, they focussed on the supervisory alliance and sought regular feedback from supervisees.

In their study, Cook and Ellis (2021), found that 77.7% of supervisees were receiving inadequate supervision and 62.3% were currently receiving harmful supervision. Much like the alliance in practitioner and client work, the supervisor/supervisee alliance when ruptured can ruin the relationship if left unchecked. Thus, Watkins (2021) informs us that 'opening up discussion and collaboratively processing the rupture – has been identified as central to increasing the likelihood of successful repair'. Just as the practitioner endeavours to create a culture of feedback with clients, so should the supervisor with the supervisee. Wilson et al.'s (2016) meta-synthesis findings illustrate that it is important that the supervisor was both able to provide feedback and receive it themselves. It is essential that supervisees feel safe with their supervisors, and that they are allowed to make mistakes, and be encouraged and nurtured by their supervisor to discuss such issues, difficulties, and challenges that they face in their client work. Said another way, supervisors must create psychological safety in which the supervisee feels safe to voice concerns about aspects of supervision that they are unhappy with.

Patton and Kivlighan (1997) and Reese et al. (2009) found a strong positive relationship between supervisor and supervisee alliance, and practitioner and client therapeutic alliance. Thus, it makes empirical sense to utilise a measure of the supervision alliance for the supervisee to provide feedback on the process and outcomes of supervision. The Leeds Alliance in Supervision Scale (LASS) (Wainwright, 2010) is the supervisory equivalent of the alliance for the practitioner–client relationship. The LASS is administered by the supervisor towards the end of the session and asks the supervisee about their experience of the relationship, the approach to supervision, and if the supervision session met the supervisees needs. The purpose of the LASS is to promote feedback and discussion about the supervisory alliance so it can be used as an effective component of clinical supervision. Ultimately, the desire and willingness to solicit and take feedback from supervisees may also be indicative of humility on the part of the supervisor, a characteristic that has been demonstrated to underpin effective supervision (Jones & Branco, 2020; McMahon, 2020; Watkins et al., 2019).

Conclusion

Supervision is an integral part of the practitioners' development, however, in its current practice format the effectiveness of supervision on client outcomes is weak. We propose that the modern twenty-first century practitioner and supervisor use objective means to assess their effectiveness, in doing so, conveying an attitude of humility and openness to learning more about their individual growth needs. Using these data, the supervisor can support the supervisee to find their limitations and areas where further development is needed. Using this information can further support the use of DP. The next chapter will provide a simulated case study demonstrating how a supervisee engages in DP supported by the supervisor, their outcome data, and linked to a client case vignette.

References

Alfonsson, S., Parling, T., Spännargård, Å., Andersson, G., & Lundgren, T. (2018). The effects of clinical supervision on supervisees and patients in cognitive behavioral therapy: A systematic review. *Journal of Cognitive Behavioural Therapy*, *47*(3), 206–228. https://doi.org/10.1080/16506073.2017.1369559

Bambling, M., King, R., Raue, P., Schweitzer, R., & Lambert, W. (2006). Clinical supervision: Its influence on client-rated working alliance and client symptom reduction in the brief treatment of major depression. *Psychotherapy Research*, *16*(3), 317–331. doi:10.1080/10503300500268524

Bernard, J. M., & Goodyear, R. K. (1992). *Fundamentals of clinical supervision*. Boston, MA: Allyn & Bacon.

Bogo, M., & McKnight, K. (2006). Clinical supervision in social work. *The Clinical Supervisor*, *24*(1–2), 49–67. doi:10.1300/J001v24n01_04

Brown, G. S. (J)., Cazauvieilh, C., & Simon, A. (2021, June). Clinician engagement in feedback informed care and patient outcomes [Web article]. Retrieved from http://www.societyforpsychotherapy.org/clinician-engagement-in-feedback-informed-care-and-patient-outcomes

Brown, G. S., Simon, A., & Foster, L. (2021, June). Clinical impact of school-based interventions [Web article]. Retrieved from http://www.societyforpsychotherapy.org/clinical-impact-of-school-based-interventions

Carpenter, J., Webb, C., & Bostock, L. (2013). The surprisingly weak evidence base for supervision: Findings from a systematic review of research in child welfare practice (2000 2012). *Children and Youth Services Review*, *35*(11), 1843–1853.

Cook, R., & Ellis, M. (2021). Post-degree clinical supervision for licensure: Occurrence of inadequate and harmful experiences among counselors. *The Clinical Supervisor*, *40*(2), 282–302. doi:10.1080/07325223.2021.1887786

Davis, E. D., & Curthbert, A. D. (2016). Humility and psychotherapist effectiveness: Humility, the therapy relationship, and psychotherapy outcomes. In *Handbook of humility*. London: Routledge. ISBN 9781315660462

Ellis, M. V. (1991). Critical incidents in clinical supervision and in supervisor supervision: Assessing supervisory issues. *Journal of Counseling Psychology*, *38*(3), 342–349. https://doi.org/10.1037/0022-0167.38.3.342

Goldberg, S. B., Babins-Wagner, R., Rousmaniere, T., Berzins, S., Hoyt, W. T., Whipple, J. L., … Wampold, B. E. (2016). Creating a climate for therapist improvement: A case study of an agency focused on outcomes and deliberate practice. *Psychotherapy*, *53*(3), 367–375. https://doi.org/10.1037/pst0000060

Grossl, A. B., Reese, R. J., Norsworthy, L. A., & Hopkins, N. B. (2014). Client feedback data in supervision: Effects on supervision and outcome. *Training and Education in Professional Psychology*, *8*(3), 182–188. https://doi.org/10.1037/tep0000025

Hawkins, P., & Shoet, R. (2012). *Supervision in the helping professions* (4th ed.). Maidenhead: Open University Press.

Hook, J. N., Watkins, C. E., Jr, Davis, D. E., & Owen, J. (2015). Humility: The paradoxical foundation for psychotherapy expertise. *Psychotherapy Bulletin*, *50*(2), 11–13. Retrieved from https://societyforpsychotherapy.org/humility-the-paradoxical-foundation-for-psychotherapy-expertise/

Jones, C., & Branco, S. (2020). The interconnectedness between cultural humility and broaching in clinical supervision: Working from the multicultural orientation framework. *The Clinical Supervisor*, *39*(2), 198–209. doi:10.1080/07325223.2020.1830327

Kühne, F., Maas, J., Wiesenthal, S., & Weck, F. (2019). Empirical research in clinical supervision: A systematic review and suggestions for future studies. *BMC Psychology*, *7*(1), 54. https://doi.org/10.1186/s40359-019-0327-7

Mahon, D., Brown, J., & Simon, A. (2021a, July). The relationship between session-to-session change on a therapeutic alliance measure and outcome of treatment for short term psychotherapy [Web article]. Retrieved from http://www.societyforpsychotherapy.org/the-relationship-between-session-to-session-change-on-a-therapeutic-alliance-measure-and-outcome-of-treatment-for-short-term-psychotherapy

Mahon, D., Brown, J., & Simon, A. (2021b, August). The relationship between measures of alliance and outcome in psychotherapy lasting more than five sessions [Web article]. Retrieved from http://www.societyforpsychotherapy.org/the-relationship-between-measures-of-alliance-and-outcome-in-psychotherapy-lasting-more-than-five-sessions

McMahon, A. (2020). Five reflective touchstones to foster supervisor humility. *The Clinical Supervisor*, *39*(2), 178–197. doi:10.1080/07325223.2020.1827332

Minami, T., Davies, D. R., Tierney, S. C., Bettmann, J. E., McAward, S. M., Averill, L. A., … Wampold, B. E. (2009). Preliminary evidence on the effectiveness of psychological treatments delivered at a university counseling center. *Journal of Counseling Psychology*, *56*(2), 309–320. https://doi.org/10.1037/a0015398

Nelson, M. L., Barnes, K. L., Evans, A. L., & Triggiano, P. J. (2008). Working with conflict in clinical supervision: Wise supervisors' perspectives. *Journal of Counseling Psychology*, *55*(2), 172–184. https://doi.org/10.1037/00220167.55.2.172

Nissen-Lie, H. A. (2020). Humility and self-doubt are hallmarks of a good therapist. Retrieved from https://aeon.co/ideas/humility-and-self-doubt-are-hallmarks-of-a-good-therapist

Patton, M. J., & Kivlighan, D. M., Jr. (1997). Relevance of the supervisory alliance to the counseling alliance and to treatment adherence in counselor training. *Journal of Counseling Psychology*, *44*(1), 108–115. https://doi.org/10.1037/0022-0167.44.1.108

Rast, K. A., Herman, D. J., Rousmaniere, T. G., Whipple, J. L., & Swift, J. K. (2017). Perceived impact on client outcomes: The perspectives of practicing supervisors and supervisees. *SAGE Open*, *7*(1), 1–10. https://doi.org/10.1177/2158244017698729

Reese, R. J., Usher, E. L., Bowman, D. C., Norsworthy, L. A., Halstead, J. L., Rowlands, S. R., & Chisolm, R. R. (2009). Using client feedback in psychotherapy training: An analysis of its influence on supervision and counselor self-efficacy. *Training and Education in Professional Psychology*, *3*, 157–168. https://doi.org/10.1037/a0015673

Rousmaniere, T. G., Swift, J. K., Babins-Wagner, R., Whipple, J. L., & Berzins, S. (2016). Supervisor variance in psychotherapy outcome in routine practice. *Psychotherapy Research: Journal of the Society for Psychotherapy Research*, *26*(2), 196–205. https://doi-org.jproxy.nuim.ie/10.1080/10503307.2014.963730

Snowdon, D. A., Leggat, S. G., & Taylor, N. F. (2017). Does clinical supervision of healthcare professionals improve effectiveness of care and patient experience? A systematic review. *BMC Health Services Research*, *17*, 786. https://doi.org/10.1186/s12913-017-2739-5

Son, E., & Ellis, M. V. (2013). A cross-cultural comparison of clinical supervision in South Korea and the United States. *Psychotherapy*, *50*, 189–205. doi:10.1037/a0033115

Wainwright, N. (2010). *The development of the Leeds Alliance in Supervision Scale (LASS): A brief sessional measure of the supervisory alliance*. Clinical Psychology thesis, Leeds University.

Wampold, B. E., Kim, D. M., & Bolt, D. M. (2006). Therapist effects in psychotherapy: A random-effects modeling of the National Institute of Mental Health Treatment of Depression Collaborative Research Program data. *Psychotherapy Research*, *16*(2), 161–172. https://doi.org/10.1080/10503300500264911

Watkins, C. E., Jr. (2020). Psychotherapy supervision: An ever-evolving signature pedagogy. *World Psychiatry*, *19*, 244–245. https://doi.org/10.1002/wps.20747

Watkins, C. E., Jr, Hook, J. N., Owen, J., DeBlaere, C., Davis, D. E., & Van Tongeren, D. R. (2019). Multicultural orientation in psychotherapy supervision: Cultural humility, cultural comfort, and cultural opportunities. *American Journal of Psychotherapy*, *72*(2), 38–46. https://doi.org/10.1176/appi.psychotherapy.20180040

Watkins, E., Jr. (2021). Rupture and rupture repair in clinical supervision: Some thoughts and steps along the way. *The Clinical Supervisor*, *40*(2), 321–344. doi:10.1080/07325223.2021.1890657

Whipple, J., Hoyt, T., Rousmaniere, T., Swift, J., Pedersen, T., & Worthen, V. (2020). Supervisor variance in psychotherapy outcome in routine practice: A replication. *SAGE Open*, *10*(1), 1–11. https://doi.org/10.1177/2158244019899047

Worthen, V. E., & Lambert, M. J. (2007). Outcome oriented supervision: Advantages of adding systematic client tracking to supportive consultations. *Counselling and Psychotherapy Research*, *7*(1), 48–53. doi:10.1080/14733140601140873

Wrape, E. R., Callahan, J. L., Ruggero, C. J., & Watkins, C. E., Jr. (2015). An exploration of faculty supervisor variables and their impact on client outcomes. *Training and Education in Professional Psychology*, *9*(1), 35–43. https://doi.org/10.1037/tep0000014

Chapter 13

Simulated Psychotherapy Case Study for the 21st Century Practitioner and Supervisor

Daryl Mahon

Abstract

The application of therapeutic theory to routine psychotherapy practice is a complex area, and needs to be done by a competent and well-trained practitioner. The case study is recognised as a valid method to illustrate the processes of therapy and how theoretical knowledge can be applied to practice scenarios to bring about change. This simulated case study illustrates the application of therapeutic variables based on evidence based relationships and responsiveness. A therapist and client-simulated case illustrate these applications, and an accompanying narrative elucidates the role these play in the therapeutic encounter. Finally, the chapter describes how some of the issues identified in the case study as practitioner deficiencies can be used to inform a deliberate practice (DP) training regime supported by supervision and the use of data. In doing so, this chapter builds on the previous chapters in this book and provides a picture of how the twenty-first century practitioner and supervisor can use data to better inform their individual, and collective work, with the ultimate aim of improving expertise in order to increase client outcomes.

Keywords: Psychotherapy; case study; theory to practice; cultural humility; pluralistic therapy; deliberate practice; twenty-first century practitioner

Evidence Based Counselling & Psychotherapy for the 21st Century Practitioner, 159–174

doi:10.1108/978-1-80455-732-720231013

Chapter Learning Outcomes

(1) Assess the application of various therapy variables to a case study.
(2) Reflect on how these factors can be applied to your individual practice.

Background to Case

Shaun is a 37 year old Black gay male, working as a college professor at a local university who first sought help due to feelings of anxiety and low mood. Shaun reports increasingly feeling more anxious and suffering from dark cloud handing over him. There has been lots of debates going on in the university regarding Black Lives Matter and this is making Shaun feel on edge. Coupled with this, Shaun feels the need to be guarded about his sexuality as he has had a bad experience in university when a professor mocked him for being gay in front of the entire class. Friends of Shaun are pressurising him to 'come out' and that he should be proud of his sexuality, something Shaun feels very nervous to do, this tends to cause friction with his friend, with Shaun becoming angry. Sleep is becoming increasingly more difficult, and daily tasks are much more burdensome due to a lack of energy and some loss of interest. Shaun reports using alcohol almost daily to help him cope with the anxiety and stress, and he is becoming worried that it may impact his employment in the university.

Initial Assessment

Shaun attends his first appointment at a local mental health outpatient clinic, with John, a White cisgender male therapist. The initial clinical assessment is generally 90 minutes in duration, used to gather data and a background on the presenting problems, and where indicated, to administer a battery of assessment measures of various types.

T: Hi Shaun, great that you could make it today, I have been looking forward to meeting with you. I know when we spoke on the phone last week that things did not seem to be going so good for you? I'm curious to hear a little more about how you have been doing?

C: Yeah, I'm just on edge a lot, my anxiety levels are quite high, and my mood can be very low on some days. I'm finding it hard to relax, and sleep … I suppose I'm doing a bit more drinking than usual too.

T: Sounds like you are going through the mill. Has anything occurred in recent times that you can identify as contributing to how you are feeling?

C: Well, there's a lot of conversations about racism happening in the university, conversations that absolutely need to be happening. But, I guess they are making me feel anxious. My department is staffed with predominantly White people, and they keep looking to me for answers …

T: Ok, there is a lot going on for you. It feels like you are experiencing pressure from your colleagues to help make sense of what is happening in society? It seems to me like you are doing your best to manage all this added anxiety and fluctuation in your mood, and alcohol is helping you do this?

C: Yes, yes, exactly … I guess that I am also really like I cannot be myself, you know. Like as a gay Black male I am feeling very isolated. I can't let others know about my sexual identity, when I was a student, I had a professor mock me in front of the entire class …

T: It's a very lonely place to be. You really want to be able to express who you are, but there's this fear of being seen, perhaps an anxiety of being stigmatised and discriminated against. Correct me if I'm wrong, but I have a sense that your previous experience as a student and the professor humiliating you is impacting how you are feeling with this current situation …

C: Yes … Shaun's eyes begin to fill with tears …

Comments

As this short narrative illustrates, the practitioner is using the initial assessment to gather information, build rapport, and attempt to understand Shaun's presenting problem. At the same time, we can see here that the practitioner is expressing empathy first at a low level (sounds like you're going through the mill), and then at a more advanced level by touching on feelings (humiliation by the previous professor) just outside of Shaun's consciousness, and how this may be impacting on how Shaun is currently feeling.

T: Shaun, in order for us to set some goals and provide you with an effective treatment experience, I have some assessment questionnaires that I would like you to complete, is this ok with you?

C: Sure.

T: Evidence tell us that using these assessments as part of a structured process to identify problem areas, and then to provide individualised treatment based on this information is more effective and produces better outcomes for clients. In addition, we use these measures to track how you are doing on a weekly basis and if the treatment approach that we decide on together is working …. Does this make sense to you?

C: Absolutely, I like that the service thinks about treatment in this way …

T: So, it fits with your ideas about how treatment should be conducted?

C: Defiantly, yes.

T: Ok, perfect. I'm going to ask you to first fill out this form, no need to write anything as it can be filled out online on this tablet, it's called the Outcome Questionnaire-45 (OQ-45) and it will help us to make sense of some of the experiences you are having, including symptoms, and how sever you are experiencing these problems across various parts of your life .... The second questionnaire that I will ask you to fill out explores the type of treatment experience you would like, your goal, the style, modality, and who and how this treatment is delivered. I have several ideas myself on what way we can work together, however, it is important that we collaborate with each other to get the best fit for you, am I making sense?

C: Yes, sure, but can you help me understand the purpose of these questions a bit more ...

Comments

Several things are noteworthy in this short exchange. Firstly, the practitioner is working from an evidence based practice perspective and using what we called clinical expertise from the tripartite model in Chapter 2. The practitioner was aware based on Shaun's initial explanation of his distress that anxiety, depression, and substance use were areas of concern. This helped the practitioner make the clinical decision that the OQ-45 (a measure of global distress) would possibly be the best tool to use as it covers each of these areas, and has lot of evidence supporting its psychometric properties and effectiveness as an ongoing measure in clinical practice. The measure assesses three core domains, symptom distress, interpersonal relationships, and social role, while also asking about critical items such as suicide, substance use, and anger at work or school.

In addition, clinical expertise is also being utilised by incorporating a questionnaire on preferences, the Cooper Norcross Inventory of Preferences which is another questionnaire that has supporting evidence while also operationalising the third part of the tripartite model, client preferences, characteristics, and culture. Finally, the practitioner is beginning to build treatment credibility and outcome expectancy by explaining the process and evidence for using these questionnaires to inform the treatment experience. As we can see this was done confidently, and with verbal fluency, which itself is integral for building expectancy. It is important to not only provide the rationale for the use of such measures, but help the client understand their meaning and implications, so sitting with the client as they fill out the measures may be needed for some, especially with preference questionnaires.

T: Thanks for completing these questionnaires Shaun. I notice that the score on the OQ-45 is quite high, 120, generally we consider anything under 64 to be low. If I can just clarify with you, your answers to the questions indicate that symptoms and social role are where much of your distress is and to a lesser extent some issues with interpersonal relationships, does this match with your experience?

C: Yes, this fits with how I am coping. My low mood, and anxiety are what troubles me mostly, in the context of my employment with a little difficulty in my interpersonal relationships because of the pressure I feel, so I'd say it's pretty accurate.

T: Perfect. I guess before we start to discuss goals and a possible treatment plan, I would like to discuss your response to the preference questionnaire. What strikes me most at this stage is that you have a preference for a Black female practitioner, and I guess, I'm not (*practitioner attempts a little humour*).

C: Shaun, smiling at the joke, yeah, I suppose if it's possible, I think I might feel more comfortable with a Black female …

T: That makes perfect sense Shaun. Unfortunately, we are a small clinic and the two practitioners fitting those demographics are on leave for the Summer. What we can do, is we have a Black male practitioner who may be available, or I could refer you to another clinic?

C: hmmm, I suppose, we have already begun this process, let's see how we get on together for now …

T: Ok, sure, but, if this changes please let me know, I won't be offended, I just want the best experience for you. I would like to explore some of the other preferences that you have based on your responses. You seem to have a strong preference for exploring the past, with no other strong preference for, or against …

C: Yes, I think shining a lens on my past experiences may help me.

T: My general way of working would be based on behavioural modification and also work around cognitive restructuring of negative core beliefs, which I think may be especially helpful to work with here.

C: I was rather hoping to speak about these issues, I have never spoken about it before.

T: Ok, maybe we can meet in the middle? How about in session we can examine these past experiences, but, with a view to having a more active approach at a future point that will involve some exercises outside of the session …

C: That sounds like something I can get onboard with, yes.

T: Great, our time is almost up for today. But before we get into the work I wonder if we can take a bit of time at our session next week to tease out your goals a little more to inform your treatment plan?

C: Sounds good.

T: Just one final thing before we finish up. If you can take two minutes to fill out this 4-item questionnaire. Research tells us that client outcomes are improved when there is an agreement on the goals and tasks, and the methods to be used, in the context of a supportive relationship. This 4-item questionnaire asks about these factors, so I will ask you to fill it out at the end of each session, it will act like a GPS, by letting us know if we get off track. Just to say, I'm not looking for top marks I'm far from perfect, so I'd be surprised if you score it perfectly all the time. Please do let me know, even something that you think may be no issue worth mentioning, I'd still like to hear about it, so as I can be in a position to offer you the best treatment experience possible.

Comment

There is a lot to unpack across these interactions between Shaun and the practitioner. Let's consider the first and last interactions, in this sequence. The use of the outcome measure (OQ-45) and the use of the alliance measure together you will remember is what we refer to as feedback-informed care. That is, monitoring the outcome (global distress) and process (therapeutic alliance) on an ongoing basis in order to capture in real time, the clients experience, and to improve cases at risk of negative outcomes. In addition, systems like ACORN can be used to help practitioners and supervisors think about their developmental needs and to inform DP exercises.

With regard to Shaun's preferences, the first point to note, is that the practitioner was aware of some of the research around cultural matching and how this can improve outcomes when it is a preference of the client (evidence based practice and clinical expertise). It is not always possible to provide the client with the type of preference that they have, and when this cannot occur, it is essential to enter a 'negotiation' as we have seen in the above scenario with the treatment style. Once again, it is important for the practitioner to stay within their individual scope of practice, as such, this may mean making a referral or indeed negotiating with the client an approach that both can agree on, and are happy with. Finally, it is integral that the rationale for measures and their use are articulated to the client, and with measures of the therapeutic alliance that the practitioner communicates humility and a willingness and openness to hear feedback from the client. The therapeutic alliance as we see in this part of the scenario is being developed early on through a negotiation on the approach to be used, and the tasks of therapy.

Session 2

T: Shaun, I know we spoke at our previous session about using today to inform your treatment plan and goals for therapy. I'm curious if you had any time to reflect on these since we last met?

C: Yeah, I guess I would like to stop feeling so anxious around my colleagues, and for my mood to improve, and I'd like to stop drinking too.

T: Ok, I know we briefly spent time discussing the role of your sexuality in this last week?

C: Well, yes, I just want to be myself and not to feel judged or afraid to let others in …

T: Let me just take a moment to clarify this. What I'm hearing is that your goals for treatment are to start to feel better emotionally, to express yourself as you see and experience yourself, and to develop a healthy lifestyle and way of coping that will enhance your relationships and work life?

C: Yes, I want to live a happy fulfilled life.

T: Yes, of course you do. I'm wondering, I know we spoke about spending some time on exploring past experiences, I'm aware that some of your goals seem to involve changing aspects of behaviour, how do you see that occurring in the context of your treatment goals?

C: Well, at the moment, I feel a bit overwhelmed and don't feel ready to jump head on into taking action right now, but certainly I do want to try it …

Comments

While the process of beginning to think about goals occurred in the previous session, this session explicitly focussed on it, with Shaun and the practitioner collaboratively identifying and naming goals, and possible methods to work on these. You will see from the exchange that the practitioner reflected Shaun's goals back as positively valanced goals as opposed to what Shaun wanted to give up/ change. At the same time, the practitioner introduced the idea of how Shaun wants to go about achieving these goals, and in doing so the practitioner identified that Shaun while willing to begin the process was still somewhat ambivalent and possibly in the contemplation stage of change. These exchanges, along with the information gathered at the last session was enough for the practitioner to begin to make a case conceptualisation and to provide a rationale for the presenting problem.

T: Shaun, it seems to me that your past experiences of being humiliated and mocked in front of your fellow students has had a huge impact on you emotionally, and on your sense of self. So big was this impact, that you have carried it with you all these years, fearful to let others into your life, and see you for who you really are. Your method of coping is to internalise things and attempt to manage them yourself. These experiences seem to be more pronounced presently due to the context of your work, and the wider societal issues happening with racism. This is making you even more anxious, especially when it comes to interacting with your colleagues, and friends, your symptoms of anxiety and low mood are coming from this pressure and you are attempting to do the best you can to manage this, including using alcohol. However, the alcohol use seems to be stopping you from facing some of these issues head on, and in doing so, the avoidance is paradoxically making things somewhat worse. I'm curious to hear what you think of my hypothesis?

C: When I hear it said like this, it makes perfect sense, yes …

T: I think we are on the right track to. And I believe exploring these issues and how you manage them, and what ways you use to cope with problems can be a first step for us in therapy, with some behavioural exercises added a bit later when you feel ready, is probably a good way to address some of these issues, especially the avoidance and to lead a more healthy emotional life.

Comments

We can see in this interaction that the practitioner has provided Shaun with a rationale for the presenting problems which is acceptable, including identifying the internalising coping style that Shaun uses and how this impacts on him by becoming quite self-critical and not expressing emotions in an adaptive way. At the same time, there is a set of techniques/rituals discussed that are consistent with the rationale of the problem. Another rationale might look quite different, perhaps someone working from a biomedical perspective may explain Shaun's presenting problems in terms of diagnoses that have a biological underpinning with a treatment approach based on medication. The key here is that the explanation and treatment are culturally acceptable to Shaun, and not that the explanation is the scientifically correct one, per se.

C: I'm quite surprised, I didn't think that I would be able to connect with a heterosexual guy.

T: I don't see a gay male Shaun, I see another person, just like me, who is doing their best to make it in a world that can sometimes be cruel.

Comments

This is a critical juncture in the course of therapy thus far. Shaun has opened himself up to be vulnerable about his initial feelings of working with someone of a different sexuality. This was not only an opportunity for the practitioner to respond through cultural humility, but the actual response provided by the practitioner who was attempting to convey unconditional positive regard, was experienced as a micro-aggression by Shaun.

C: I see …

T: Tell me more about your past experiences, I think starting to process these emotions now is a good place to begin.

C: Maybe next week.

T: We still have 20 minutes left, how would you like to use your time?

C: Let's call it a day, I'm feeling a bit off.

Comment

The practitioner senses that something has changed in the energy between him and Shaun, we'll recall from previous chapters the idea of alliance ruptures, specifically a withdrawal rupture. The practitioner thinks this may be a good opportunity to finish the session by checking out his initial hunch by using the alliance measure.

T: Sure, if that's what you would like to do. Just before we finish up, I wonder if you can score the alliance measure so we can take the temperature of how we are doing? I have a sense that something has changed between us, but I just can't put my finger on it, I wonder if you can help me understand …

C: Give it here …

T: Ok, great … you seem to have scored the measures a great deal lower this week, thank you for your honesty. Can you help me understand what went …

C: What went wrong?, what went wrong?

T: Um, yes …

C: (*Shaun getting more vocal and angry*), I am not just like you. In fact, I am nothing like you. How dare you try to compare my life and experiences with yours, and see me just like you. You are just like all the rest of them, am I safe around anyone at this stage? (*eyes beginning to tear up*). I wish I never came here at all (*voice rising*) you have been no help to me …

Comments

Shaun has strongly voiced how he is feeling and a clear alliance rupture is apparent. In comparison to the previous type of rupture, this is a confrontational rupture. This is a critical point in the therapeutic alliance and if not managed well can often result in client dropping out of therapy. Many practitioners can struggle with these types of ruptures, but without addressing it, no meaningful therapy can occur. As we see the alliance measure being filled out is one way to identify the rupture, or in this case what I would call a multicultural rupture, and to begin the process of cultural humility.

T: Shaun, thank you for bringing all these to my attention. You are correct, my response to you was invalidating, and for this I am very sorry. I attempted to show that I don't see you as fundamentally different, but in doing so, I invalidated your experience of being a gay man in an often oppressive heterosexual world. Shaun, I hear how angry you are towards me, and the impact this has had on you … I hope that you can give me another chance, a chance to respond differently, more supportive towards you …

C: I guess, it wasn't intentional …

T: I also sense how hurt you are by my response. I have let you down, you put your trust in me, and in many ways I have recreated how you feel around colleagues, and perhaps even in some way, the deep hurt you felt when mocked by your college professor, the very issues you came to see me about and wanted to work on.

Comments

This scenario demonstrates advanced rupture repair skills, as well as advanced levels of empathy. The practitioner validates Shaun for broaching the subject, and does so in a non-defensive manner. The practitioner takes ownership of the rupture by acknowledging their part and seeks to re-establish the alliance by seeking another opportunity to be more supportive. The practitioner also demonstrates advanced levels of empathy, by empathising with the negative feelings directed towards them and the reasons for these feelings, while also addressing the underlying hurt and emotion that may have been out of awareness. Finally, the practitioner linked the rupture to experiences that Shaun has outside of therapy in his interpersonal relationships and reason for seeking therapy.

C: Yes (*now crying*), I just …

T: I know you spoke previously about finding it difficult to express your feelings …

C: It's, they feel mixed up, I can't always capture them …

T: Where on your body are you experiencing them?

C: My stomach.

T: If they had a voice, what would they say …

Comments

We can see in this exchange that the practitioner having previously responded with depth empathy is building on this experience in the here and now by encouraging emotional expression (another variable) with the emotions that are now conscious. As Shaun's coping style tends to be internalised the practitioner felt that being a little more direct with regard to the expression of emotions was warranted. We join the session at a later point after Shaun and the practitioner have processed some of the emotions.

T: You know Shaun, I feel much closer to you …

C: How so?

T: It's like I know you in a different way, you have trusted me with your inner most feelings … feelings that have not been easy for you to expose, even to those you consider to be most close to …

C: True, and I guess that's why I'm coming here, to be able to do that with the people that I care about …

T: I wonder if exploring our relationship can help with that. I know earlier I seemed to have brought up quite a strong reaction in you? I have a hunch that this may be a familiar response that you have to your friends when the topic of your sexuality comes up?

Comments

In this short passage, the practitioner in the first instance demonstrates congruence by expressing their inner thoughts and feelings in relation to the clients. As we can see from the response, Shaun is open and ready to receive this message, and to see how it links to his goals for therapy, that is, the practitioner has used congruence in relation to Shaun, in doing so the practitioner and Shaun are activating the alliance. The practitioner then moves onto using immediacy, by drawing on the here and now example of the interaction that caused the rupture. The practitioner wonders if this is how Shaun generally responds to those he cares about when the issue of his sexuality is broached, and what learning can occur by examining this, again activating the therapeutic alliance.

Supervision and DP

Let us know move on to examine what can be learned by the same practitioner from using data-informed supervision, and DP based on both micro- and macro-areas for improvement. In the following supervision scenario, we will demonstrate how learnings from one case can be of assistance and help us identify areas for further development. You will recall that the practitioner in the previous dialogue used a feedback-informed treatment system, much like the ACORN system my colleague Dr Jeb Brown provides. Therefore, supervision, as in the previous chapter, can be data informed. In the scenario below, the practitioner has been working with a data informed and DP supervisor for the last 12 months, and has seen their outcomes improve. In this supervision session, the practitioner brings the case of Shaun up for consultation.

S: It's been about two months since we last met, how have you being getting on with the DP exercises that you have set as learning goals?

P: Really good actually, I've had a few difficult encounters with distressed clients just this week, and the alliance rupture–repair and advanced empathy exercises have really helped build my capacity to responding to clients. Not only that, but those counter-transference exercises that we were working on last year, to help stretch my emotional regulation capacity seem to have helped.

S: Great to hear .... Have you an agenda for today's session, you mention that you have had a few difficult cases these last weeks? Would you like to begin there, or have you something more pressing?

C: Yes, I had a challenging session last week, a new client, we'll call him S. Actually, the alliance rupture exercises that I have been using DP on worked really well, so I'm happy with that. It's more so, I suppose I feel quite bad, I missed some important markers about the client's sexual identity, and invalidated the client who is gay, and is struggling with keeping that part of the identity from work colleagues. There is anxiety, low mood, and some alcohol use as methods to cope, and a previous bad experience with someone in authority where S's sexuality was mocked in front of others. So, yeah I'm just reflecting on this.

S: I know that we have being using DP to practice eliciting lower alliance scores in the early sessions, did you manage to have any luck with that this time?

P: Actually, yes, well the first session no, as the alliance was scored perfectly, but after the incident S did mark the alliance down, so that was good, and I then got to repair the rupture using the new skills.

S: Great, I wonder if exploring what happened might be beneficial to our learning?

P: I guess that I was trying to convey unconditionality, but it seems that I invalidated S by suggesting that I view him just like me, as another human.

S: Ah, yes, could have been experienced as a micro-aggression by S.

P: Exactly, I noticed something was off, the knowledge around the withdrawal rupture was really helpful, so thanks for that.

S: Sure. I suppose we are getting into the area of cultural identity here, I have a hunch that exploring some of your data may be helpful, what do you think? Would you like to open up your outcome system?

P: Absolutely.

S: I'm just mining the data here and breaking it out by demographics, and I'm noticing that your effectiveness with ethnic minorities is somewhat lower than with White people, and your dropout rate is also higher, is this something that you were aware of?

P: Well no, not my effectiveness, I hadn't thought to examining the data from this perspective, I kind of thought that my dropout rate might be a little lower, but I wasn't sure.

S: Just looking at your initial intake alliance score, it is perfect and seems to remain perfect throughout the entire treatment duration, yet outcomes are lower and in some cases we can see some clients have a marked deterioration in their global distress levels before dropping out.

P: So, some of my clients are actually getting worse while with me, before dropping out.

S: Yes, research tells us that about 8–10% of clients deteriorate while in care, although this can be higher for some practitioners. Do you have any initial thoughts on what needs to change?

Comments

We see here that the supervisor is helping the practitioner, in a supportive non-judgemental manner to mine the data to look for themes and patterns of where alliance scores many indicate something is amiss, and using outcome data from global distress scores to support this. The supervisor also normalises that lots of practitioners experience drop out and clients who deteriorate while in care, while also seeking to find out if the practitioner has any idea why the data are illustrating these patterns.

P: Well, not really, I guess working within the diversity space can be difficult, I didn't receive much training in this area during postgrad school, and I suppose I don't tend to have many relationships with anyone other than my White middle class circle. I suppose that I don't like to see people as different, my professors in grad school were quite humanistic and I have carried this belief with me, even though I like more directive approaches too.

S: This makes perfect sense, and it is something I see quite a lot, with lots of my supervisees. I like to refer to it as being culturally encapsulated, both in our therapy training, modalities, and lack of diversity in studies, but also based on how and where we were raised, our socio-economic background, and how we continue to socialise, especially if we don't mix in diverse circles.

P: I suppose this makes me feel a little better, I have been beating myself up a little.

S: I have an idea. We can't say for sure what is happening with your work with ethnic minoritised clients, however it is clear based on the data that your outcomes are worse with this population of people. And while the data cannot tell us the why, the one piece of information that we do have from your last client, is that you missed important cultural makers when they occurred. Although we can't say that this is happening with all clients, I think we need to consider this as perhaps a deficiency in this area until we have information to say otherwise. Agreed?

P: I suppose when I hear you say it that way, then it makes sense to me.

S: I feel learning the multicultural orientation with a key focus on cultural humility will be a good DP exercise to start with. I have some simulated videos that we can use for you to begin skills acquisition with, it's the same process that we were using for the DP exercises in alliance rupture–repair and advanced empathy. We can watch the video in supervision and I can provide some feedback on your responses, and you can build on this in your own time using a diverse range of videos, I have several other types. As with some of the other exercises, you can record yourself practicing and we can review the recoding's in supervision and assess how you are progressing, how does this sound?

Comments

It is beyond the scope of this chapter to illustrate the DP drills. However, you will find the processes involved in the multicultural orientation in Chapter 9. You will also recall from Chapter 11 that I spoke about five processes involved in DP. These five processes can be seen in the above dialogue. The practitioner is setting goals just beyond their ability, the supervisor is designing the DP regime and providing expert feedback (more knowledgeable other, MKO), there is repetitive rehearsal of the specific cultural orientation skills outside of therapy hour, and there is a continuous assessment of performance by the practitioner and supervisor by observing the recordings, and later on by examining if outcomes are improving in the data.

DP Framework

When thinking about beginning DP, the following variables in Fig. 2 depict where to direct your energy and the magnitude of the effect size of each. It is not a prescriptive model, but rather a guiding framework that practitioners can use to identify their idiosyncratic needs based on a thorough examination of their effectiveness in differentiated areas of practice. Practitioners should be conscious of the effect size of each variable, and aim their DP training in areas that demonstrate to be most impactful. Using data and getting a coach or supervisor who is an MKO is a necessity to support clinical decision making. For many, this may seem an overwhelming task, and in some ways it can be if not done correctly. DP takes time and effort, and some variables may be much more difficult to progress in. As such, I recommend only choosing one variable at a time, and directing your energy on this aspect exclusively, setting up DP drills that consist of behavioural rehearsals, and direct feedback, in addition to monitoring your outcomes in these specific areas.

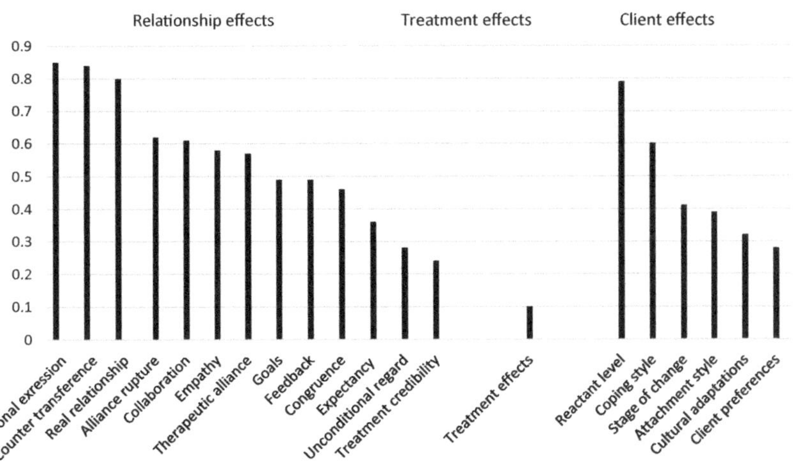

Fig. 2. Contextual Deliberate Practice Model.

Conclusion

This chapter has provided a simulated client case example of the application of many of the common factors and variables discussed throughout this book, bringing what can be very abstract concepts into the clinical domain. The twenty-first century practitioner now has at their disposal, the use of data that can inform their clinical work by reducing the risk of negative outcomes and early drop out from treatment. However, the use of data goes beyond the clinical hour and can extend into the supervisory relationship where supervisors can support the practitioner through mining of data, to establish areas of deficiency for further development, and by using these data and clinical information to support and develop DP exercises.

Index

Printed and bound by CPI Group (UK) Ltd, Croydon, CR0 4YY

12/08/2025

14717773-0002